MEDICINAL HERBS AND NATURAL REMEDIES

The best healing foods and herbs in the mediterranean diet and tradition – Recipes on the preparation of natural syrups

ROBERT FRANCISCO DIAMOND

ISBN: 978-1-80169-319-6

Table of Contents

Chapter 1

Traditional Mediterranean Medicine and Medical Plants

In ancient civilizations, everything is a symbol; the Myth has the same the function of the Symbol is to transmit a Reality to us superior, untranslatable through the formulation alone But while the symbol is figurative, the Myth uses it instead of a story, of a tale beneath which lies a profound concept.

The Symbol connects two objects or two situations through thought analog that is through the similarity; this way of seeing reality is common in societies traditional.

Myth is a means of transmitting a reality transcendent that is placed in an eternal present and neunderlies immutability, it can be considered as a matrix unconscious arising from the images of the unconscious collective; the Myth is an archetype that unites all human beings, from every place and every time.

Indeed Jung, in his studies and through the observation of the patients of him could see the similarity of some images from the unconscious in different people that they had nothing in common with each other and did not have knowledge about the image that emerged; therefore not having to do with cultural baggage and with personal experience of the person, it could be considered an archetypal image, part not of the individual unconscious but of the collective unconscious, which is the common substratum a all human beings, regardless of race, from gender and age.

An image that frequently appears between archetypal figurations of the unconscious is that of the tree, or the miraculous plant in general, in the past Two types of Medicine were used: a direct, immediate one, which causes healing through intent, or the use of pure will, which is the medicine of Christ or of Asclepius, the other who works about the knowledge of world and the correspondences between man and the various kingdoms of nature.

The latter is based on the law of similitude that characterizes the medicine of Hippocrates, of Paracelsus (in part) as well as the Chinese one, which they use herbs, acupuncture, and massage, natural and attuned methods with nature but less direct than the other method.

In direct medicine, the pure and desireless will it is exercised either by the healer through the simple laying on of hands, by word or ritual, or from the sick person himself who works in itself a profound transformation, a healing of the spirit as well as of the psyche followed by the body healing. Plato states,

"The doctor heals more with his soul than with his hands ".

The Latin proverb states: "Mens Sana in corporate Sano";

but we can also affirm the opposite:

" Corporate healthy in men's Sana "because the disease originates at the level thin, only later, when it condenses on the level material manifests itself on a physical level."

The ancient Greeks attributed the origin of medicine to god, Asclepius, thus demonstrating the divine art of healing the man.

According to the common tradition, Asclepius was the son of Apollo and Coronis, and at first, he was only one hero, albeit gifted with overtime powers; subsequently assumes divine dignity in the myth.

The emblem of Asclepius was a rod wrapped around it one or two snakes: the animal symbolizes wisdom in genre, and in particular the wisdom of man-medicine.

This symbolism is also linked to the fact that in the temples of Asclepius used snakes were bred as a healing tool.

Snakes also had a function in Egypt sacred; in fact, the eyes of the blind were made to lick from the snake's tongue.

The snake is also a symbol of power: we find it on the head of the kings of Egypt, as an ornament and symbol together.

In the Caduceus, the two coiled snakes represent the eternal duality between good and evil, the spirit and the matter, positive pole and negative pole, the rod in the middle represents the god's ability to balance them two forces.

The Caduceus also represents the power to reconcile each other different elements; that is, water, earth, fire, air; for this, it is a a symbol that often occurs in Alchemy. The Caduceus came attributed first of all to Hermes Trismegistus (he who is three times grande), the mythical ancestor of magical art traditional understood as a noble synthesis of universal knowledge in all its applications.

The term Hermeticism derives from the name of Hermes Trismegistus to indicate initiatory knowledge.

Greek mythology then took up the myth of Hermes that of it drew the legendary messenger of the gods Hermes, then become the Mercury of the Romans. Mercury is the messenger of the gods and is, therefore, the mediator of their will with the men.

He knows how to stand next to mere mortals and receive theirs desires, their needs; he was commissioned by Zeus to assist men in their transition from life to death, accompanying them to the abodes of Hades.

It is named for this Hermes. Psychopomp: the companion of souls.

As a messenger of the gods, he moves with the swiftness of thought, and also his shoes, like the helmet and the Caduceus, are equipped with wings. The symbol of the snake is also found in the Christian tradition.

An ancient depiction represents the virgin Mary who she crushes the snake with her foot: the strength of the spirit that dominates over instincts; in fact, the snake in this case represents matter.

In the Indian tradition, however, the snake symbolizes the kundalini, the sleeping serpent, located at the base of the thorn dorsal, which once awakened releases the extraordinary energies inherent in the human being.

This energy, however, can lead both towards the divine and towards craving and thirst for power, depending on whether you are rise upward or descend into the bowels of the earth snake is considered a symbol of medicine because the Sick people must make themselves a body and a soul to get well new, or leave the old skin as snakes do with every change. Hermes is also the cheat, in mythology it is the imaginary being, often identified in an animal who plays colossal pranks on men.

In fact, Hermes is identified with four different animals placed at the four cardinal points: to the North, it takes the form of a snake, in the south it has the shape of a wolf, in the east, it is an ibis, while ad west takes the form of a monkey.

He represents duality, the good versus the evil, the wise and the fool, the serious and the joker, the destroyer of worlds and the savior of humanity.

He belongs to our world, and at the same time, he is not part of it.

He is a creator, a joker, a keeper of truth and history.

Hermes represents the double reality we live in, the positive and negative, yin, and yang. It is also the child that we hide in us, self-centered and eager, attentive, capricious, and spiteful.

Due to its dual conjoined nature, Mercury is designated as a hermaphrodite; now hers is defined as feminine his body and masculine spirit, now the opposite.

Another aspect of Mercury's contradictory nature is that of being young and old at the same time: the the senile figure of Mercury attested by archaeological excavations it undoubtedly brings it closer to the old Saturn, young as it is Mercury is often referred to as a son or a child.

Ermete Trimegistro is the acknowledged author of the Table Smeraldina is the description of the natural laws of matter and the universe. Egyptian tradition has it that Thoth, like Hermes to the Greeks, revealed the Hermetic arts to the men. One of these arts is Alchemy. Thoth means "truth." and also, Ermeth in the Coptic language means True. Table emeraldine is considered 5000 years old; the phrases contained in it have been found in many papyri

The Egyptians are encoded in the emerald tablet expressions that make it a mighty formula for achieve spiritual transformation and accelerate the evolution of the human species through achievement of the highest states of consciousness.

It would be molded into a single rectangular block of crystal green, or pure emerald, with letters in low relief of a strange, unknown, similar alphabet to the ancient Phoenician.

On the tablet, it is written: *"It is true it is certain and very true that what is below is as in high, and how that which is above is like that which is below, to perform the miracle of one thing.*

You will separate the earth from fire, the subtle from the thick. Here lies the strength stronger than any strength because it will win everything subtle and will penetrate everything that is solid. In this way, the world was created for this reason, I was called Ermete Trimegistro, owner of the three parts of philosophy around the world ".

Latin alchemy holds the whole mystery in an allegorical key Christian, the creation of Adam is assimilated to the work alchemical, since as God drew Adam out of the mud, so the alchemist draws the Philosopher's Stone from a base matter.

Through alchemical operations the vital force of man and all substances up to reach Quintessence. Man is lead who it must be refined, perfected to become gold before the light of the Universe.

Ovid's "Metamorphoses" begins with the narration of the origin of the universe, at first a shapeless and indistinct mass later separated and modeled in the four elements from the cosmic alchemist: "Before the sea and the earth and the the sky that covers everything, unique and indistinct, was the aspect of nature throughout the universe and they said it Chaos, shapeless mass and confused, nothing but an inert weight, a mass of conflicting germs of things badly combined ... And as far as there was the earth, and the sea and the air, unstable was the land, not navigable the wave, the air devoid of light: nothing could keep its shape, each what contrasted the others, since in the same body the cold it struggled with the heat, the damp with the dry, the soft with the hard, the weight with weightlessness, a god, and a more benign disposition of nature, healed these contrasts: he separated from heaven the earth, from the earth the waves, and distinguished the sky from the thick air pure. And after having untangled and released these things from the shapeless mass, he dissociated the seats; he united them in a whole agrees.

The fire, imponderable energy of the celestial vault, shot put, and yes settled in the highest region.

Immediately below, due to its location and lightness, the air, the earth, and denser absorbed the larger elements and remained pressed into low from its own weight. The water, fluid, occupied the last spaces wrapping everything around the solid mass of the world "

Chapter 2

The humoral theory

One of the leading figures of Traditional Medicine Mediterranea is certainly Hippocrates of Cos (460 BC).

He belonged to a family of doctors who, according to the tradition, descended directly from Asclepius (the god of medicine).

The set of books attributed to Hippocrates goes under the name of Corpus Hippocraticum.

The Corpus works can be divided according to their contained in different groups:

1) Books with ethical content

2) Books by clinical and pathology

3) Surgery books

4) Books of obstetrics, gynecology, and pediatrics

5) Anatomy books and physiology

6) Books on therapeutics and dietetics. Anatomy was not very thorough from the school of Cos.

We had notions of osteology, especially regarding the structure of the bones of the skull, vertebrae and ribs. Heart and brain were known as the main ones morphological characteristics but not the real functions herbs the Hippocratic school provided for their use of hellebore and Scilla (cardiotonic and diuretics), Hyssop as an expectorant, Opium, la Mandrake and Belladonna as narcotics and analgesics, Mint as a stomachic ... However, knowing the main groups of medicines, the school Hippocratic used them little as he put away a lot confidence in the self-healing capacity of the human body.

Hippocrates is remembered above all for the wording of the humoral theory in which he pointed out the fact that there are four fundamental moods present in Human Body; the mixture and the proportion between these four bodily senses of humor determine the constitution individual.

In reality, this theory has much more origins ancient; however, its paternity is attributed to Hippocrates.

The four basic body humor are:

Blood, Bile, Phlegm, Melancholy.

The four moods were then combined with the four elements *"Fire, Water, Earth, Air,"* these unalterable, original elements

and immutable, therefore eternal. These four elements have allwithin them a temperament that distinguishes it from Others: Fire has heat as its natural attribute, Air has dryness as a natural attribute, water as an attribute natural has the humid and finally the Earth whose natural attribute is the cold.

However, each element, while retaining the property the dominant background may have other characteristics secondary.

For example, if in an organized substance the hot and secondarily, the humid one will say that the substance in question is hot in the first degree and humid in the second.

In the vegetable kingdom, the plant consists of this Mood, i.e., hot-humid, will be a plant anti-inflammatory and soothing such as Mallow, which Dioscorides also speaks of in the "Matter Medica ":" Soothes the intestines, plus fresh leaves

chewed and pulped applied with honey weld the scars and help bee and wasp stings and whoever applies the fresh Mallow mush and oil cannot give they are stung. The boiled leaves cure burns and the Sacred Fire ".

Furthermore, the four elements were divided into two classes

In one, we find the Fire and the Air, which together constitute the "forming form," while Water and Earth is the "material."

So Fire and Air represent the energetic part while Water and Earth the material substratum.

In addition to the Fire was recognized as the "specialty." energy, "movement" to Air, "quality" to Water of matter, and the Earth, the "quantity."

The yellow Bile corresponds to the Fire with the attributes the liver produces it; the Blood corresponds to the Air it has its seat in the heart and represents the vital spirit of Water corresponds to the Phlegm that resides in the head, while the Earth corresponds to melancholy or black bile. That the spleen produces it.

Later Galen, in his treatise *"De temperament is"* connected each bodily mood to a specific temperament, namely: Yellow bile corresponds to the Bilious temperament, i.e., choleric and impulsive in which liver functions prevail; it is the passionate temperament par excellence.

To the Blood corresponds the temperament.

Sanguine; cheerful and expansive with a predominance of circulatory system. Black bile corresponds to Melancholic or Nervous temperament, or sensitive e susceptible, with a predominance of functions.

Finally to the Lymph or Phlegm corresponds the Lymphatic temperament; lazy and dreamy with the predominance of the lymphatic system. Every organism it contains in itself blood, yellow bile, phlegm and melancholy, in fact, Hippocrates writes: "This is what constitutes the nature of the human body and which creates the disease and health.

There is indeed health when these moods are the right ratio of mixing, strength, and quantity, and therefore the mixture is perfect. On the contrary, there is a disease when one of these humor is in defect or excess, or separating in the body is not combined with the whole rest. "(Of the nature of man).

These Humor are based on various organs of the body: in the

spleen black bile-Earth, in the liver the yellow bile-Fire, in the head the phlegm-Water, in the heart the blood-Air. Galen (130-200 AD) whose teachings they had huge following throughout the Middle Ages and in renaissance, he practiced for a long time the profession a Rome under Marcus Aurelius becoming a physician of the gladiators. He took up the Hippocratic teachings that they were largely abandoned in previous centuries the numerous works must be remembered: "Ars Medica." and "De temperaments."

He takes up the Hippocratic Theory of Humor by matching each mood a certain temperament: if the prevailing mood was Blood the the subject was defined as sanguine; if it was yellow bile, it came defined choleric, if Phlegm predominated, it was said to be phlegmatic; if Black bile prevailed instead; it was defined as melancholic.

Purification of bodily humor could be implemented in the following ways:

1) Through the stimulation of two or more organic functions simultaneously, for example, skin disease due to blood intoxicated provides for the purification of kidneys, liver and the connective system.

2) In other cases, it is possible to resort to stimulation of a single function, as in the case of kidney stones.

Purification can take place spontaneously, through spontaneous seizure, that is, through the access of fever, sweating, vomiting, diarrhea; or it can be induced through the use of active substances.

From the Platonic tradition, Galen derived the idea of the vital Breath or pneuma regulator of human functions, subdivided in three different categories depending on its location:

psychic that has its seat in the brain and nervous system, vital that resides in the heart, the vegetative function in the liver.

He also took an interest in the eye of mammals, lending particular attention to the crystalline and to that affection which takes the name of cataract, concluding that the crystalline is a fundamental structure for the vision, so much so that when a person is affected precisely from cataract, which veils the lens, loses the ability to to see.

He believed in the medicinal use of opposites: contrary contrariis curantur; for example, he supported the effect Beneficial of Pepe to warm the patient also nearly 500 simple substances of vegetable origin among which the most famous the Picra (bitter purgative based on Aloe) and Hera (colonquintide-based sacred purgative).

Returning to Hippocrates, his medicine comes commonly considered a positive medicine and rationalist, in reality, if it is partially opposed to the forms of medicine put into practice until then for practice accurate clinical observation not only through sight, but also touch, hearing, smell, and taste, and then reasoning which, by integrating these elements, allows you to evaluate, judge, and formulate a prognosis, on the other hand, yes integrates with relationship-based cosmological medicine macro-micro cosmos considering man as part integral to a greater Whole.

In the treatise "On the Sacred Disease," one wanted to see one

the manifestation of a scientific-looking positivism modern: "he has nothing more divine, more sacred than others, but nature and source are the same as those of other diseases ". But then he continues the speech saying:

"comes from the same influences as the others, that is to say from this that comes and from what goes, from the cold, from the sun, from the winds that change continuously and never interrupt the their action. These things are divine, so it dictates the disease has no characteristic that confers it a more divine character, but all are divine, and all are human beings ". Thus depriving one of the sacred characters disease, it returns it to all.

Sacred because through it we can evolve, because the disease it is not just the consequence of the attack of a bacterium, or by a harmful substance, but it is also and above all the spy that one is lost contact with the part deeper than oneself, with its central core, of consequence even if the illness is not a pleasant thing, a sometimes represents the last attempt of our inner voice to make us understand that something is wrong, that we have to change something in our lives and try to rediscover the profound meaning.

Nowadays, the disease is considered an unfortunate one hiccup, something to hide and referred to to be ashamed, and modern medicine is often made of analgesics and tranquilizers, antibiotics and cortisone, medicines to suppress the symptom and suffocate it, methods that do nothing but hide the dust under the carpet instead of eliminating it, it's a kind of medicine that instead of solving the problem at the root tends only to make the disease chronic, as if to say: *"Live a long and sick "*.

The disease is fought as something external and of strangers from us, instead of as Hanemann affirmed, "The the bacterium is nothing; the soil is everything. "In reality, the disease it should be seen as a combination of factors, in part resulting from the interaction with the outside, in part from

our genetic and psychological predispositions; Moreover seen from a more spiritual point of view, the disease is a failure awareness and a. times eliminate the symptom it just means turning off the light, instead of the sick person were empowered and yes treated as such could evolve on its own "thanks" to the disease.

However, despite its limitations, its validity must also be recognized of official medicine, especially in acute and severe cases that require immediate relief and effect; while that so-called "alternative."

It is more suitable for the prevention and mild acute and chronic ailments and medium entity; however, in my opinion, the two medicines do not they must be seen as alternatives, but they must be considered complementary, with two different ways of dealing with the disease, but both with their own dignity, so instead of fighting each other they should work together to have a broader view of disease and the sick person.

Unfortunately, lately, we are witnessing a new "Hunt for witches ", in fact, many try to throw mud on medicine natural making it pass for not serious, or for crooks stuff.

Natural medicine has its limitations, this is beyond doubt, but it has the great merit of considering the person, not just the disease, and to also consider the patient's experience, what he thinks, how are his relationships with others, and to seek the origin of disturbance, both on a psychological level, because diseases are often there indicator of internal discomfort, both physical, without going to suffocate the symptom, but if anything going back to the organic cause when a person suffers from an allergy, usually the doctor officer prescribes antihistamines and cortisone, which do not resolve absolutely nothing, they can be useful only in acute cases.

For example, when a person is suffering from an asthma attack, but temporarily and in the lighter cases as in the case of a rhinitis, it would be appropriate to change the diet in fact allergies are connected to the liver, according to Chinese medicine; therefore, eating in a lighter way and eliminating certain foods can be greatly reduced or even resolve the allergy altogether. I had the experience even on myself, in fact, I have seen that every time I exceed the eat, or that I eat cured meats or foods loaded with toxins the next morning, the allergy is triggered while on a diet slight allergy disappears.

Returning to the discourse on Hippocrates and traditional medicine in Cos, the place of origin of Hippocrates, there was a

Temple dedicated to Asclepius. In fact, at the time of Hippocrates the medicine, exercised by himself, he has neither forgotten nor denied its origins, in the "Hippocratic Corpus," can be found therein fact connection of medicine to the divine and the existence of a esoteric teaching: "I swear on Apollo doctor, on Asclepius, on Hygieia and Panacea, on all the gods and goddesses I take as witnesses, that I will absolve, according to my strength and my ability, the oath and the following commitment:... I will communicate the precepts to my children, to the children of my teacher, and the disciples linked to a commitment and an oath to medical law, but none more ... I will spend my whole life and practice my art in innocence and purity .... Whatever I see or hear in the company during the exercise of my functions, or even apart from that exercise, I will not spread what should not be disclose, and I will consider it a secret"

Very little is known about the archaic practice of medicine in Greece: There may be some fascinating suggestions offered by the allusions present in the Homeric poems, which recall a world in which elements magical, mythical traditions, empirical use of herbs for the purpose Therapeutic and surgery coexisted in mythological poems we often find hints on the use of herbs, which they have a partly real and partly fabulous use, as in case of the Moly herb narrated in the Odyssey.

-When Ulysses and his companions arrived on the island dawn Sea, where the sorceress Circe reigned, this one being the enemy of humanity, she transformed all Companions of Ulysses in swine. Ulysses was saved thanks to a talisman was given to him by Hermes: a white flower from black root, called Moly, which only the gods can recognize and collect.

- Another episode narrated in the "Metamorphoses" narrates that Jason, to conquer the Golden Fleece, had first to face of the tests imposed by King Aetes, such as that of yoking two bulls spitting flames on the plow. Medea, priestess of Hecate, to help him she gave him the Crocus saffron-colored Caucasian, which would protect him from the flames spit by bulls. The Caucasian Crocus who helped create the Mysterious fame of Medea is the poisonous Colchicus, considered by the ancients as the most effective remedy for gout.

After all, the Crocus in the Greek religion has always been associated to the female figure; in fact, Pallas Athena wore a colored peplum saffron during religious rituals, and also the garments of the "ark too," the orse, or the child priestesses, were of the same color.

Also, in the Greco-Roman tradition Hymenaeus, or the protector of the marriage bond is wrapped in a cloak of this color.

The Crocus, like all plants connected to the Great Mother, has an ambivalent meaning, on the one hand, inferior and on the other solar, symbol of life and death, a symbol of a principle that everything generates and welcomes everything at the end of the cycle in its womb cosmic.

After all, this duality is confirmed by phytotherapy; in fact Pliny wrote that the Crocus had a property fecundating, but at the same time, it could be second Dioscorides, a powerful poison.

Crocus sativus or saffron used in the kitchen, once upon a time known more for its medicinal properties than for those culinary; Dioscorides advised him how antispasmodic, while Arab medicine prescribed it as emmenagogue. In Italy, the species of Crocus from which it is derived saffron is widespread, especially in Abruzzo, and is considered one of the best in the world.

Returning to the story of Jason and Medea, Jason succeeded in this way to tame the bulls and force them to plow the field, but King Pete not wanting to respect his pact, she refused to give him the fleece.

However, the king had imprudently confided in Medea, the she whom she accompanied Jason and the Argonauts to the sacred precinct of Ares where the fleece was, guarded by a hideous dragon; but Medea managed to configure him by spraying him with drops soporific from freshly cut Juniper twigs.

Also, the episode in which Jason asks his wife, Medea, to extending the life of the now dying father sees the Goddess of night use herbs for her magical arts: "They were missing three nights for the crescent moon to close in a circle perfect.

When the moon shone full and came all-around a contemplating the earth, Medea left the house wearing one the dress was undone, barefoot, bare hair spread over her shoulders, and she went with wandering steps to the silent silence of the midnight ... Stretching its arms towards the stars, it turns three times on herself, three times she spreads water on her hair river, she thrice she opens her lips and howls and knelt down she on the hard ground she says:

"Night, most faithful keeper of the mysteries; golden stars, that with the moon you succeed the flashes of the day, and you Hecate from three heads that you know what I try and come to give strength to the chants and the arts of wizards; Earth that you supply mages with powerful herbs, and you breezes and winds and mountains and rivers and lakes, gods all of the forests, gods all of the night, attend me!"

Thanks to you, when I want the rivers to return between the astonished banks at the springs, I make the agitated sea still, I wave it motionless for spell, clouds I chase, and clouds gather, I send the winds away or else I call them, I make my throat explode by reciting formulas to the vipers, I uproot and move the stones, the oaks, the woods, I order to the mountains to tremble, to the ground to bellow, to the shadows to go out from the sepulchers... Now we need juices because of the life of a old, regenerated, repaint, and go back to the flourishing years of youth.

And you will give them to me, for not for nothing do the stars have winked, not for nothing, pulled by the neck of winged dragons, here a chariot! "And a chariot descended from the sky was there at wait for her.

She climbed on it, and as soon as she had stroked the hills harnessed and with her hands, he shook the light reins; it was she carried up, and under her, she saw the Tempe tessera, and she did drop dragons in certain regions.

He scanned the herbs that were on the Bone, the herbs that were there high Pelion ... and the ones she liked she tore from their roots or she cut them with a curved bronze sickle. She also plucked grass vivifying in Antèdone, a herb not yet famous for transformation of the body of Glauco.

And now nine days and nine nights they had seen her search all campaigns on the chariot with the winged dragons. she returned dragons had been touched only by the perfume: yet they lost their skins of ancient animals. she Returned she stopped outside front door ... with her hair down like a bacchante, she goes around of the two altars, on which the fire burns; she soaks torches from the many tongues in pits black with blood, and so she drenched them alight the fire of the altars; and she purifies the older man, three times with the flame, three with water, three with sulfur, and a filter in the meantime powerful, in a pot, boil, and dances whiten and It bubbles where it cooks roots cut in the valley of Emonia, with seeds and flowers and spicy juices ... When with these things, and with a thousand others without a name, the stranger had prepared what was needed for the gift promised to dying; with a very dry branch of a peaceful olive tree, she stirred the all mixing the top with the bottom ".

The complex and ritualized use of herbal drugs is incorporated in a system that is both magical and pharmacological at the same time and derives from the ancestral culture of the Mediterranean, founded on cult of the Great Mother.

Medea is one of the last mythical representatives of the image-priestesses of the Great Mother, who in the myth of Argonauts, she appears as an ally of male heroes, bearer of the terrible secrets of Earth, Night, and Darkness.

Medea is the custodian of ancient wisdom, actual rituals, she utters words of power, spells, and formulas magical, she alters the nature and destiny of people and things she chooses special moments for the implementation of rituals magical: at midnight, on a full moon night, in the moment in which three stars shine, especially; the relationship with the moon is typically feminine, connected with cyclicality and the regular and harmonious changeability and adaptability of The night is also invoked through Hecate, the dark one Triform Goddess, where everything that is converges dark, nocturnal, celestial, and underground at the same time.

Medea uses herbs of power, both magical and pharmacological, these two aspects in ancient times were inextricably linked together. She flies in the sky at night up a chariot pulled by winged dragons/snakes; therefore, she confirms herself the celestial, nocturnal aspect of Medea while the winged serpents that carry the sorceress-priestess in flight or carry on a journey underlie the use of state-inducing techniques and substances ecstatic-shamanic.

Medea, in addition to the rigorous implementation of a complex ritual, she uses herbs (not stated in the Myth, aside Aconite, also known as the Devil's Grass for its poisonousness.

In fact, it contains various alkaloids that act on the system nervous resulting in death from cardiac paralysis or Respiratory herb, used for the evil of witches and witches, like the mythical episode of Medea On the Metamorphoses, Ovid narrates that Aconitus was formed from the coagulated slime of Cerberus and that Medea prepared one potion to kill Theseus) and parts of animals and others substances; these parts are not important in themselves, but for theirs symbolic and metaphorical value:

- Owl wings; the owl is, therefore, a nocturnal bird of prey also heavenly and flying.

- Werewolf entrails; the werewolf represents the reciprocal human-animal transformations, typical of all ancestral shamanic procedures, moreover the werewolf is connected to the Night and the Moon and therefore to the Feminine.

- Frost collected on a night of the full moon, a symbol of the Waters celestial and condensed by the Cold Snakeskin; the skin is the molt, the change and the renewal in the orderly regularity of biological cycles, the the serpent is the messenger of the crawling mother Earth from darkness to light

- Long-lived deer liver: indicates the perfect relationship between Mood production and youth-longevity; (the liver is the center Producer of Blood and heat) - Head and beak of a crow spanning nine centuries, more complicated symbol;

crow, like the deer, is a Melancholy animal, but unlike this, it feeds on corpses, as the owl is " psychopomp "or accompanying souls of the dead in Hades. All mixed with the peaceful Olivo.

Another interesting aspect that many of the popular fairy tales once narrated about witches are very similar to the passages of Ovid in the Metamorphoses, yet the grandmothers are unlikely who lived in the countryside knew Ovid, as they did not they knew the illiterate peasant women burned at the stake from the inquisition only for using herbs and rituals to aim to heal someone, in fact once in the countryside it was often these simple women who lived in harmony with nature, and they knew its secrets and virtues the role of healers.

Among the male figures in Greek mythology, that of Asclepius for its direct link with medicine.

According to the Greek poets Hesiod and Pindar, Asclepius would be lived shortly before the Trojan War.

He himself would have participated in the expedition of the Argonauts in search of the golden fleece, sharing with all the heroes, his expedition companions, his art medical, son of Apollo and the mortal Coronado, he possessed like other heroes of antiquity (Dionysus, Hercules ...) a half-human and half nature.

He was raised by the centaur Chiron who taught him medical art.

In addition to treating the sick, Asclepius had the faculty of resurrect the dead, and because of this, Hades, the god of the underworld, fearing for the prosperity of his kingdom, he complained to his brother Zeus.

These, believe that in fact, the order of the world was threatened by Asclepius, he struck him with his thunderbolt, and at the same time, Asclepius passing through the fire ascended to the role of divinity.

Sacrificed because of his love for him humanity, Asclepius thus deified was invoked as savior of men, and as a god of health and of medicine.

Asclepius and Christ have often been compared to each other.

Both possess the two natures, the divine and the one human, both manifested their love towards men and died for allowing them to become immortal.

Even in their artistic representation, they are compared to point that a statue of Asclepius in the fourth century AD it was co-merged with that of Christ.

Asclepius' preferred method of healing was direct and immediate, which originally was practically the only method was then progressively replaced by methods intermediates through the use of herbs, massages ... hand as knowledge of the Principle faded.

However, Asclepius is also remembered for an episode less noble.

-A legend tells that when Hercules wounded hades descended into hell to capture Cerberus, he called to his bedside Peonio, son of Asclepius, for him to cure him.

Petronio healed him so well that his father was attacked by one crisis of envy that did not bode well then Hades rescued it by turning it into a plant beautiful, the Peony, the "rose without thorns."

With large solitary flowers, pink, red, and even white, and come on fleshy fruits.

Peony was considered an effective remedy against madness. "If you tie a weed fool around the neck Peony, you will see him come to his senses immediately. "The root instead, it was recommended to treat epilepsy in children.

Roots and petals fought against asthma and gout Indeed, the Peony is also called gout rose.

Returning to mythology and its link with medicine is possible

to affirm that the mythical event represents a stratification of meanings inherent in various realities; that medical-biological is typical of some figures;

we could indeed say that all mythical figures are related to medical-biological aspects, each in a particular way.

Among the great goddesses, Artemis emerges first of all, fused with the Diana of the Romans, Goddess of the night, of the wild hunt, of the unattainable virginity of Nature she not yet tamed by crops.

But Artemis-Diana is also a collector of herbs, the preparer of drugs, donor to human beings of the healing powers of herbs. In the courtyard of a patrician house from the Napoleonic era is the copy of an image of Diana the Huntress who could represent part of the foundation of ancient physiology, with some reference to the pathology.

The Goddess stands with her right arm bent backward that slips an arrow from the quiver, hanging from the her right shoulder; the quiver appears full of darts; the left hand instead of carrying the bow, she is leaning down on the head of a deer crouched at her feet; on Diana's forehead, it shines a silver crescent moon. The Greek term for the bow is suggestive: "toxin," which is the basis of all the terms that have a what to see with "poisonousness," "toxicity," in effect "Toxicon" indicates the poison in which the arrows are dipped; the link between archery and poisonousness is very ancient, original, ancestral.

Chapter 3

The knowledge of poisons

The knowledge of poisons corresponds, always ancestral, with knowledge of substances in general and their activities pharmacological.

Indeed the term itself has a complex origin: the term "drug" is connected with an Indo-European ancestral entry with multifaceted meaning: a deadly spell.

The quiver hanging from the right shoulder symbolizes the gallbladder and the arrow the yellow bile; the golden color confirms the hypothesis. Also, many biliary diseases do physically highlight with pain and discomfort at joints of the right shoulder and right side of the neck. According to Traditional Chinese Medicine, there is a established connection between right scapular area and gallbladder, and according to Traditional Mediterranean Medicine, the part the gallbladder, and for rule right of the human body first, it undergoes the imbalances due to yellow bile;

it accentuates in young people, in irascible subjects, and on everyone during the attacks of anger, during the summer and eating and drinking "Hot" foods and beverages (such as meat and wine).

The arrows, sharp and thrown far, constitute the yellow Bile's perfect allegory, making all more penetrating, light, and diffusive body moods. Arrows also indicate hot and dry drugs, ruled by Fire, and which they give to the body lightness, fluidity, warmth. They favor fluidization of the mucus, the opening of the obstructions, the desperation of Cold clots and "consume" the Moisture. The Bile yellow is the hottest, sharpest, most subtle, and penetrating of the Four Moods.

On the head of the Lady of the Woods (Silvia in Latin, in English Silver is silver, lunar metal, aqueous and feminine-Cold par excellence) is affixed to the Crescent Lunar, silvery-white shining.

It represents the raw whiteness of the "Waters Lunari "Cold and coagulated typical of mucous membranes and gods more or less pathological mucus. Phlegm is formed in head favoring "head" affections such as sinusitis, the head is the source of body fluids e of sensitivity.

Sensitivity is in fact attributable to the Moon, the star of fantasy and intuition, the feminine, and the tides.

To decongest the mucous membranes of the upper airways in case of rhinitis and sinusitis, Thyme can be used. an excellent balsamic plant, expectorant and antiseptic, useful in case of asthma, bronchitis, and whooping cough.

Thyme acts under its heat as a stimulant and accelerating on the mechanisms that regulate the response immune system dynamizes circulation and stimulates the lymphatic system.

Hence a strong plant is shown in the elements Earth and Metal (according to Chinese medicine).

It is also useful in urinary infections and rheumatism chronic (Water element).

It is a yin plant with some yang elements that the Greeks considered Thyme symbol of courage and resourcefulness; while the Romans do they inhaled the sweet fragrance to fight melancholy.

It is the favorite plant of bees, in fact, the medieval ladies they used to give their knights a scarf on which it was embroidered a bee flying around a twig of Thyme to instill courage in them.

Philochorus of Athens, soothsayer and profound connoisseur of the rites report that it was the Thyme that fed the flame of the gods more ancient sacrifices, the "nephàlia," where one abstained from every libation of wine.

Its very name explains the sacrificial use of the thymus Greek "thymos" which derives from the verb "thymiào," which means: "I burn like perfume." It was translated into the Latin "thymus." that has given the name to the two main species, "Thymus vulgaris" and "thymus serpillum ".

The latter was called so because he wrote Pliny, *"meanders, which happens especially in the wild species in rocky soils, while the cultivated one does not crawl but grows in height up to a palm "*.

Since the name recalls snakes, in ancient times, it was said that was effective against reptile bites, especially reported Pliny: "against cancer (a snake so called because his skin was speckled with similar spots with millet grains) and against the scolopendras, both of earth and of sea and the scorpions need to boil the twigs and leaves in wine ". It is said that fairies love him, so who wants to meet them should prepare an infusion with hers inflorescences. In the Renaissance, it was recommended cooked in wine, for asthmatics, but also to treat irritation of the the bladder, eliminate tapeworms, heal from poisonings and promote menstruation.

It was used dry, pulverized, and mixed with clay as a toothpaste and gum disinfectant.

Essential oil with properties is extracted from Thyme antiseptic and antispasmodic.

It was once recommended as a suitable drug to cure orally, typhus and dysentery or inhaled, tuberculosis, the bronchitis and whooping cough.

- Taking up the discourse on the representation of Diana, in

to her left, a deer is crouched.

Against the bad melancholy, one of the substances used since from the most remote antiquity was the Coral, which it has an unmistakable "deer antler" shape.

Coral is made up of calcium carbonate, with relevant quantity of magnesium carbonate essential for the proper functioning of muscle fibers and for the treatment of various forms of depression.

Diana-Artemis represents the wild aspect and originating from the vital phenomenon; the forest, the environment wild, it is its seat and source of food and gods Medicaments and still today a large part of the medicinal substances derive from substances and materials coming from the uncultivated, wild environment.

Also, in Greek mythology, Artemis is the sister of Apollo, God and governor of the Medical Art; as He is armed of arc.

The Greek term for the arch is suggestive: "toxin" - poison; in fact, the arrows and the knowledge of the poisons corresponds, always ancestral to the knowledge of pharmacological substances. Artemide inspires the collection of medicinal drugs, while Apollo governs the dazzling intuition, the diagnostic genius and therapeutic therapy of the ancient physician.

The Great Mother Goddesses inspire the "Medicine Woman," educated in ecstasy that we can define shamanic, where a great (feminine) Spirit suggests to the healer the way to the health of the sick. Apollo instead holder of therapeutic and divinatory powers inspires what he is called "romancer," or "healer-seer."

A useful plant to dispel the "bad melancholy" given by stagnation of mucus is the hyssop, especially for bronchi and lungs, therefore useful in case of diseases due to excessive presence and decreased dynamics of humor such as lymph and plasma and mucositis in general, especially the sticky ones and The hyssop was also considered important in ancient times for its purifying qualities; in fact, it came used for some purification rites of lepers and of unclean.

-In the myth of Artemis also the episode of Actaeon narrated by Ovid in the "Metamorphoses" has similarities with the Yellow Bile (Liver) and Black Bile (Spleen).

"There was a valley all covered with fir trees and pointed trees cypresses, called Gargafia, sacred to Diana from the clothes succinct.

At the bottom of it, in the thickest of the woods, there was one cave, perfect, but not for human art;

Nature, with her talent, had done a job that seemed artificial: with live pumice and light tuff, she had built spontaneously a bow. On the right, a spring of transparent water thunders and glitters, with the large framed spring from a grassy ledge. Here the Goddess of the woods, when she was tired of hunting, she used to pour pure gushes over hers limbs of a virgin.

And even now, it came.

To the nymph who acts as her squire, she gives the javelin, the quiver and bow loosened; her robe comes off, that another he welcomes her in her arms; two of her remove the sandals from her feet ...

While Diana was bathing there at the usual source of her here is that Actaeon, wandering through the woods he did not know, arrived in that sacred recess. As soon as he entered the oozing cave of the spring, the Nymphs ran to arrange themselves around Diana and covered her with their bodies, but the Goddess was higher than them, she overlooked them all, from the neck up.

She didn't have arrows handy, as she would have wanted; she took the water she had there and showered her face with it avenging gush as he said these words, omen of imminent misfortune: *"And now she says she saw me without veils, if you can! "*.

She gave her head sprinkled long-lived deer antlers; she stretched the her neck, she pointed at the top of her ears, changed her hands into feet, her arms into long paws, and she cloaked her body with a spotted coat.

And she added shyness.

He fled via Actaeon, and as he fled, he was amazed that he was fast ... he only had his old mind left. What to do?

Go home, to the palace, or hide in the woods?

While he stood there uncertain, the dogs spotted him it pursues, hungry for prey, over cliffs, cliffs, and rocks inaccessible.

He would like to shout, "I'm Actaeon! Don't you recognize me?

I am your master! "

He would like to, but he lacks the word.

And the sky thunders with barks.

The wrath of Diana carrying the quiver was only satisfied when she, for the many wounds of her, she ended her life. ".

The story of poor Actaeon has been widely used by alchemists to symbolically describe the technical procedures, both from the point of view of chemical and pharmacological effects.

The Deer, an animal sacred to Diana, indicates both the Spleen and the government of the Mood elaborated by it, or the Melancholy It is no coincidence that the horns of the animal are been used, pulverized, or reduced to ashes to cure some affections deriving from the bad governance of the Mood: in the kidney stones, in osteoarticular ones; when the blood, too full of bad Melancholy becomes little smooth, poorly oxygenated, capable of congesting the spleen itself, the uterus, the renal apparatus.

If the deer represents prudence, shyness, the elusive power of passive elasticity of muscle fibers, tendons, cartilages, connective tissue, the dog represents the impetuous bravado and imprudent aggression of Fire metabolic, the prompt reactivity of the active fibers, the muscle ones and nervous.

The hunter represents unrestrained yellow bile.

Dry, fiery, raging heat indicates searing activity The mood in producing pathologies inflammatory, painful, and febrile.

The court of Nymphs, who pour water from the spring onto the sacred body of the Goddess, represent the various ways of

Phlegm, organic water, in the body. This mood is the vector of all the others, which in part compensates in part favors give the blood the liquid vehicle and regulate the presence of "white cells," responsible immunity and how much is soluble.

The metamorphosis of the hunter (yellow bile) in deer (Melancholia) indicates one of the most common processes of ancient pathogenesis: an excess of Fire, after it burns and it incinerates, dies out, loses heat and mobility therefore remains a cold and dry Earth, often dark (the ash or charred residues), which represent one of the forms of bad Melancholia.

Dogs, possible allegories of fluidifying, opening, and drugs disintegrating cold clots, attack and dismember the deer, melancholic, and splenic allegory. The spleen congested with excess mood by herself produced or processed, it hardens and swells; dogs they will "eat it" and "consume it," not a case the major remedy for a congested and blocked spleen is the Ceterach (fern), also called "Asplenon," "without spleen "; in fact, its intake" reduces "e "consumes," relieves the spleen full of residues densely terrestrial.

In fact, one of Actaeon's dogs is called Panfago, one is called Pterela (Winged-therefore light), and three they have names that recall black: Melampo, Melania, Melanchete.

As if by magic to the trained eye of the ancient physician, little by little is revealed the design underlying the description of the mythical event.

The plants that make up the sacred wood of Diana are mostly Cypresses, phlebotomists, and hemodynamics; venous stasis is caused always from a splenic and melancholic imbalance.

Chapter 4

Cypress tincture

The decoction of berries and cypress wood is used externally for counter hemorrhoids; internally it is used to combat fever, such as diuretic and for all problems of the bladder and prostate, it acts as a tonic for these organs, with a delicate disinfectant action.

An ancient recipe based on Cypress is used for counteract varicose veins, in circulatory disorders, in hemorrhoids and menopause: - You bring ten berries of Cypress in a liter of dry white wine.

It is left to macerate for two weeks, filtered and drunk a spoon, dissolved in water, morning and evening. It is also considered a general rebalancing of the venous system.

For the whole of its constituents, it has above all an action vasoconstrictor and protective of capillaries.

Cypress tincture, which can be used in infusion or decoction, is indicated for treat phlebitis, varicose veins, hemorrhoids, while the essence of the branches is antiseptic and spasmolytic, useful as a cough suppressant.

Cypress berries are rich in copper and can be used to stimulate intellectual functions (cypress derives from super: copper).

It is also indicated in spasmodic coughs and is an effective remedy in whooping cough, in cases of pertussis, tracheitis and bronchitis.

It is used in influenza, in cases of aphonia, and moles rheumatism.

It is also effective in nocturnal enuresis.

The Cypress has taken on meaning since ancient times sacred, linked to funeral rites and death.

- Ovid tells in the "Metamorphoses" that the young Cyparissus lived in the company of a large deer golden horns.

It was hot summer noon, under the sign of Cancer; the heat-exhausted deer had settled on the ground grassy enjoying the coolness of the trees. Inadvertently Cyparissus, who was playing with a sharp javelin pierced him to death desperate, he decided to die too.

And despite the intervention of Apollo, who rushed there without delay to console him, Cyparissus asked the gods for a single privilege after death: to be able to show eternal mourning changed into the tree that bears his name.

In the Far East, the Cypress evokes immortality thanks to sturdy wood and evergreen leaves.

For this reason, Taoists feed on resin and needles.

It is also said that the resin, when it penetrates the soil, produces a kind of mushroom after a thousand years wonderful, the Fu-ling, which gives eternal life.

Another mythical character that you can do with of connections with medicine is Hercules.

According to ancient authors, the Hero is the maximum expression of Melancholy; in Hercules, all the great Myths converge of Melancholy: the impurity deriving from the murder, the countless tests conducted in a state of servitude, the betrayal of his partner Dejanira - also in turn deceived, the atrocious agony in the shirt, wet from blood of the centaur Nessus, death sought on the pyre, in purifying fire, which will bring the hero to the side of the Gods.

Centaurs are mythical figures with considerable implications

medical-biological: the equine part symbolizes the Cold-Dry terrestriality of Melancholy, during the part human represents Air, Hot-Humid like blood.

Based on these considerations, we can associate the "Herculean" muscle masses of males, to the apparatus reproductive of females and therefore to the extension of the Spleen.

Certain medicinal plants such as Poplar and are sacred to Hercules Olivo, plants that improve blood circulation making the blood more fluid and flowing. And what an analogy more suggestive of a little flowing blood than that of a A dark, dense, heavy mood like the Mixed Blood is Melancholy, the "Black Blood," which generates affections varicose contributes to hypertension, promotes severe dermatosis and other affections regulated by the excess of Melancholy circulating?

Hercules, coming out of the underworld at the end of the twelfth the effort, he weaved a crown with the branches of the planted Poplar from Hades at the Mnemosyne spring (whose water allows the deceased to access the immortality of the heroes).

In contact with the air, the upper part of the leaves remained black because this is the color of the Underworld, but the part that adhered to the forehead of Hercules turned silver-white a contact with the hero's sweat.

Therefore, the popular, especially the white one, is sacred to him: the leaves' double color indicates that Hercules has accomplished his labors in the two worlds. The white poplar symbolizes the path to a new life.

Only hers was to be used during Olympic ceremonies wood for the sacrifices offered to Zeus.

Also, in another area, in the Sumerian tombs of the III millennium, white poplar hairstyles have been found in gold, which alluded to a spiritual rebirth.

The bark of the branches and the buds of the poplars, dried in the sun, in decoction, they are also antiseptic, digestive, expectorant and sweat.

They treat bronchitis, rheumatism, neuralgia, meteorism and the decrease in fever.

As for the Olive, it seems that it came from Asia Minor where it initially grew in the wild.

According to the myth, it was an Oleastro (Olea Europea oleaster) ad to arrive first in Olympia, Greece, brought by Hercules.

In Olympia, the hero set up the Olympic Games, which took place every four years in honor of his father, Zeus.

He planted on the bare hill, which he had dedicated to Cronus, a Oleaster wood is taken from the sources of the Danube, where them he had received as a gift from the priests of Apollo.

The branches with which the crown of Oleastro was intertwined to be placed on head of the victors could only be cut with a sickle gold held by a young man of noble origins.

The olive tree offers precious fruits rich in proteins, carbohydrates, minerals and vitamins A, B1, B2, and lowers cholesterol bad Another effective plant for its properties phlebotomist, vasoconstriction, and vasoprotective due in the presence of Excluloside and its derivatives an horse chestnut, the contained Triterpenes instead have an action anti-inflammatory and anti-edematous. The action of Aesculus hippocastanum takes place through the removal of liquids The name of horse chestnut derives from the use that si in ancient times of this tree in Turkey: it mixed oats the flour obtained from its fruits to administer it to blown horses.

The horse chestnut (Chestnut bud) is a remedy present among the Bach flowers indicated for those who tend to repeat always the same mistakes and fail to profit from experience, they always get involved in relationships of the same kind, destined to fail, or they experience the same symptoms without analyzing the cause their inability to learn from mistakes can derive from indifference or lack of attention a power of observation. It helps individuals hone it

spirit of observation and to become aware of present, realizing his mistakes and tracing them back, for derive useful lessons from it.

While the White Chestnut among the remedies Bach's is suitable for those who tend to ruminate too much and constantly rethinking the same episodes.

- Returning to the topic of Spleen affections, I would like to mention its functions, especially from the point of view of Chinese Medicine, which confers on this organ much more important than medicine Western today, which almost relegates it to a role secondary.

The Spleen contributes to the transformation process of the food initiated from the stomach also provides for distribution of the processed product to the various bodies a viscera for further processing. Dysfunction of the spleen will therefore lead to disturbances digestive system, poor appetite, and general weakness.

Also, since the digestive process forms the basis for Qi and Blood formation will not be satisfactory in quality or quantity. According to Medicine Chinese, if you want to tone your blood, we must also act on the spleen. The coagulation capacity is associated with a good function, while the pathological aspect is hemorrhage, therefore the inability to keep "the shape of the blood." thermoregulation of the body; for this reason, often, the coldness at the extremities are attributable to disturbances of the spleen. The spleen is also easily affected by humidity; why this does not happen. It is necessary that its yang aspect, which comes from kidney yang, works well to make liquids produced by the organism are evaporated. If this does not happen, I accumulated fluids that could cause diarrhea, swelling, or edema, especially in the lower part of the body.

In fact, Chinese Medicine states that "the spleen loves the dryness and fear of humidity ".

A harmonious spleen ensures a mass sufficiently developed and harmonious muscle; if yes is in deficit so that you will have thin and weak muscles.

From a mental point of view, the ability to concentration, thought organization and memorization is related to the spleen, its functions therefore they are expressed above all in the activities of study and work by allowing us to set them consistently and to express ourselves clearly.

But thoughts can become worries, the structural movement typical of Yi (energy of Spleen) can close in on itself, thought folds up of oneself in a vicious circle that leads to fixed ideas and obsessions. Then there is no more room for feeling and for let emotions flow freely but only for codify and analyze, which in the long run damages the Shen because the weighted Heart can no longer fly free and light. Behind this need for order and stability, there is a deep internal fear that one tries in vain to monitor.

Chapter 5
Best Remedies and recipes for diseases (syrups)

-Ceterach syrup:

Guercino polypodium (plant and root), Borage, the bark of the root of Caper and Tamerice, each 60 gr., three handfuls of Ceterach, two handfuls of Hops, Cuscuta, Maidenhair fern, Lemon balm; 3 liters of water, 1300 gr. of sugar. Drugs are boiled until the water is consumed up to about 1-liter an half, pour by squeezing, add sugar and do it cook until syrup consistency.

This remedy is especially suitable for varicose veins, i delays in healing, including of tendons a muscles, cartilage, and bone fractures, in calculus, in immune disorders in subjects swollen with heavy fluid even in simple cellulite, finally in menopause This syrup should be given in cycles short.

- Root syrup:

Celery, Fennel, Parsley, Rusco roots and Asparagus, of each 120 gr., 60 gr. of Caper roots and of Robbia, honeydew water 3300gr., 1650 gr. of sugar.

The decoction of the drugs is made in honeydew water (two parts of boiled water in one part of honey) pour, add sugar and boil again until it reaches the consistency of a syrup.

The action of this syrup, in general, is expressed on all mucous thickenings, from broncho-pulmonary ones to intestinal, renal, hepatic, and splenic ones. The obstructed liver generates the fever, the spleen favors its chronicity, the phlegm-mucus condensed in the kidney is polluted with the

bad melancholy coming from the blocked spleen, the kidneys overheat due to the clogged liver, and with the competition of these multiple causes, kidney stones are formed according to

Humoral Doctrine of Traditional Mediterranean Medicine. -*Hyssop syrup:*

90 g. of dried Hyssop, 60 gr. of polytope roots Guercino, licorice, fennel, and safflower seeds, 15 gr. of world barley and maidenhair fern, 90 gr. of raisins pitted, 10 dates and 10 dried figs, 2 liters of water, 500gr. Of Honey and 500 of Sugar.

Drugs are boiled in water until consumed half, is poured by squeezing and add the honey and the Sugar. Cook everything until you get the consistency of a syrup.

This recipe gently cleanses the chest and lungs of ailments caused by both cold and heat. The formulation allows both a rapid expectoration of the mucus and intense anti-inflammatory action.

-*Marrobio syrup:*

60 gr. of white Marrobio, 15 gr. of Licorice roots, of Guercino Polypodium, Aniseed and 13 Cotton, 60 gr. Of Celery and Fennel, 27 gr. Of Hyssop, Oregano, Maidenhair fern, Calaminta, Thyme, Savory, Farf ara, 13 gr .. of pitted raisins, 10 dried figs, 2650 gr. Of Honeydew water, 650 gr. of Sugar and Honey, 30 gr. of dust of Iris rhizomes.

The usual procedure is followed, and finally, the powder is added by Iris.

This is a more energetic version of the previous, as an expectorant and mucolytic, with tropism accentuated for the respiratory tract and affections with more tenacious and viscous mucus, therefore useful in asthma, in chronic cough and also in pneumonia and pleurisy healing.

- Cedar syrup:

330 g. of citron or lemon peel, 2 liters of water, 1 kg. Of Sugar. The citrus peel is macerated in water; then it is cooked until 650 gr. Remain, it is poured, and yes, add sugar, then cook until one is obtained syrup. It acts on the heart when due to an imbalance from cold divine torpid and suffering from palpitations, cheers a drives away the sadness, is also effective on the stomach, and emotional affections with strong somatizations.

- Scented apple syrup:

Dispel the gloomy melancholy vapors that generate anguish e

afflictions soothe the rage and rejoice.

It contains Sweet-sour but fragrant apple juice, 1300 gr. Of violet juice, of Borage and Bugloss, Rosewater, of each 330 gr., 2 kg. of sugar. Preparation: Mix I juice and rose water, sugar is added and cooked until the syrup's right consistency.

- Altea syrup:

Cleanses the kidneys of mucus-induced obstructions phlegmatic, sticky, and purulent. Promotes elimination of pus and gravel, eliminates noninflammatory heat evident soothes the burning of the urinary tract.

Ingredients: 60 gr. of Altea, 30 gr. of chickpeas reds, Gramigna, Asparagus, Hulled licorice, Grapes pitted pass, each 15 gr. Summit of Altea, of Mallow, Parietaria, Pimpinella, Plantain and Maidenhair fern of each a handful.

12/15 gr. of Pumpkin, Cucumber, Melon, Watermelon. 12/15 gr. Of Endive, Chicory, Lettuce, Portulaca, and Sorrel. 2 liters of water and 1350 gr. sugar Preparation: Yes makes the decoction of the plants until about one is consumed third of the decoction water, pour, add it sugar and cook until the consistency of syrup.

This syrup has a powerful effect anti-inflammatory, combined with a remarkable diuretic action and a disruptor of calculations. According to the humoral doctrine the Altea-Ceci couple is above all an important garrison for the fluidification of the phlegm-mucus and its expulsion in the kidney but also in the intestine and bronchopulmonary.

Bronchial mucus and kidney stones, for ancient medicine

The Mediterranean is more or less made up of the same humoral substance.

- Horseradish syrup:

Energetically cleanses kidneys and bladder, reduces stones and it expels the gravel and also promotes diuresis when it is tiny.

Ingredients: Roots of domestic and wild horseradish of each 30 gr. Roots of Saxifraga, Rusco, Ononide, Parsley and Fennel, each 15 gr. Leaves and/or tops of Betonica, Pimpinella, Ortica, Pulegio, each one handful.

Alchechengi and Giuggiole fruits, 20 of each.

Seeds of Basil, Burdock, Parsley, of Macedonia, Caraway, Wild carrot, the root bark of Laurel, each 9/10 gr. Pitted raisins, Licorice, of each 25/30 gr. 3.5 liters of water, 1300 gr. Of sugar, 700gr. Of purified honey. In the end, add 4/5 gr. of Cinnamon and 2 gr. Nutmeg Preparation: First, the decoction is made in water until 2 liters remain.

It is poured, sugar and honey are added, and it is back to cook until the right consistency.

Finally, the pulverized spices are added.

-To remove the cold and phlegmatic humidity, it is necessary use hot remedies that increase vital heat.

Among these are the generous wine (preferably red), egg yolk, raisins, pine nuts, and pistachios.

Apio (celery for moderns) has its own specific property in the root and the seeds; it is hot in the II degree and dries in the III, opens the obstructions of the veins, arteries, and gods kidneys, lightening, and cleansing.

It dissolves the "vapors" and shakes (the vapors are the gaseous part humor, and are formed when they stagnate in the improper manner in the body; generally, it is the "melancholic vapors," which cool, favor obstructions and create psychic disturbances).

Petroselinum (Parsley) is hot and dry in the III degree and possesses the same virtue in both seeds and roots.

It consumes the humidity, opens, is an emmenagogue and diuretic eliminates obstructions and extinguishes vapors.

Fennel is active both in the root and in the seeds; it is hot in the III degree and dry in the II, it cleanses the visceral organs and i kidneys from obstructions, sedate abdominal cramps; is among the safer and more powerful remedies.

Betonica is hot and dry to the second degree; it has a fluidifying effect and detergent; it helps the suffering stomach and promotes digestion; eliminates theirs from the lungs, liver, and spleen dysfunctions; it is an emmenagogue, breaks down kidney stones heal jaundice; is suitable for the treatment of all types of obstruction, whether there is a fever or not. The Hyssop is active only for the leaves, where it is hot and dry at the III grade and composed of thin and light parts; therefore, owns a lightening and cleansing virtue for dense moisture e heavy, which expels by the intestinal route.

It acts on all organs, but its maximum activity there exerts on the lungs from which it vigorously eliminates obstructions due to thick phlegmatic mucus. Given his lightening and purifying activity the Hyssop comes also used to purify environments.

Marrobio Bianco or Prassio has leaves and seeds that they are hot in the II degree and dry in the III; since it is light and bitter energetically cleanse the liver, spleen, lungs and uterus Taken with dried iris root extracts the Thick phlegm from the chest. It is administered to women who after giving birth, they cannot expel the placenta e as an emmenagogue.

The Decade (Lavandula stoechas -Labiatae) is hot and dry in the 1st degree, slightly astringent a bitter; consumes, cleanses, and frees all organs from obstructions.Join those who have coughs and inflammation of the lungs and pleura, jaundice the black bile produced by those with the spleen.

It is good for the stomach that digest badly and nausea.

The Calaminta or Nepitella, especially the Montana, have energetic fluidifying and assertive properties;

they disperse sweat from the body and consume moisture which generates edema.

They prevent any obstruction, are diuretic and emmenagogues, they cleanse from jaundice and asthma.

Applied externally, they heat the skin, provoke irritation, hyperemia, and then ulceration.

The Pulegio (Mentha pulegium-Labiatae) possesses in equal degree heat and dryness consumes dense moisture and tenacious, it favors the expulsion of viscous phlegm from lungs and melancholy from the spleen.

The Camedrio looks like a small oak, from Greek "similar to Dryad" (Dryads are the nymphs of oaks), it is hot and dry in the III degree, it thins the humidity thick and viscous; opens obstructions of major organs and is diuretic and emmenagogue. The Camepizio (Ajuga chamaepitys-Labiatae) is dry in the III and hot in the II; it acts more or less like the Camedrio; it is active in particular in jaundice and joint diseases. The Camepizio is like that named for its turpentine smell; from the Greek Camepizio-similar to pine.

The Aristolochia, especially the rotunda (Aristolochiaceae), is hot and dry to the III degree, the root is mainly active;

the seat of action is above all the brain, where it purges from putrid and sticky phlegm, it, therefore, helps from epilepsy to uterine affections, it is also anti-abortion (means goodpartum).

It particularly acts on cough, asthma and breaks down internal abscesses can lead to miscarriage.

Aloe is hot and dry in the second degree; it is astringent and bitter, intensely strengthens the stomach, especially if it was first washed (it came dissolved in water or other liquid, the filtered solution then condensed again).

Cleanses from thick and sticky phlegm and dissolves vigorously obstructions of all major organs.

It makes the blood more flowing eliminates moisture in excess and protects from rot.

In winter, the ancient doctors, instead of decoctions and syrups administered the pulverized drugs subtly mixed with Mead, and to make it so that the penetrative virtue is expressed to the highest degree towards the more distant organs, you can add a little the liquid containing the decoction or the Guajaco powder.

The decoctions prepared with this substance are suitable for limbs subjected to excessive coldness and affections sweating is induced, but only if so the imbalance is already stretched towards the surface; otherwise, if the illness is chronic and rebellious to action therapies sudorific is of little use.

In conclusion, the main action to be sought in affections of Eliza is to thin the mucus obstructive.

Mucus-thinning and expectorant drugs they have a de-blocking action, therefore also a diuretic and emmenagogue.

Obstructive mucus is the final manifestation of Mood Phlegm, Organic Water, Cold and Wet in excess o "corrupt."

The most active plants are, therefore, those defined as Warm and They have this kind of action Umbelliferae and Labiatae, finally the sudoriferous that favor the expulsion of waste towards the outside, especially when these are already in peripheral tissues and organs, such as joints and skin. Liver remedies:

A legend has it that Prometheus, after stealing fire to give it to men, he was condemned by Zeus to be chained to a rock while simultaneously an eagle ate his liver, which he grew back each time effects the liver is an extremely vital organ, which even partially removed.

The eagle is also an animal known not only for the his pride, for his keen sight; the sight according to Chinese medicine is related to the liver.

Signs of jaundice are fever and the spread of bile yellow to the skin. The simplest care is baths fresh water and body massages with oils and ointments lightening, emollient, and promoting the circulation, among these, is the Dill oil, of Chamomile and Castor oil; ointments such as Gleucino or Musteo, containing wine must and many aromatic substances, including Sweet Clover and Calamus aromatic and macerated in unripe olive oil; the container was placed in the fermenting marc.

Another ointment was Crocino, based on Saffron, and Irino a the base of Iris, Amaracino instead of Marjoram. Remedies administered internally act on the hepatic obstruction and inflammation.

With obstruction, there is no fever, while with inflammation, there is it could be. So in case of excess liver heat, they should be avoided drugs that are too hot, such as Genziana, the Enola, the Aristolochia, and the Centaurea minor; they are indicated instead of the affection that occurs from the obstruction.

The root of Enola is suitable for the type who thinks too much (excess spleen) and physically does not work enough, since the lungs are on the borderline between spirit and matter, it is obvious that the person will somatize especially here.

The root of Enula is, in fact, indicated for asthma, chest catarrh, limp stomach, and intestinal obstruction.

The fourth part of a sprig is used by adding some wine.

The plants that cure excess liver heat are instead of the Cold-Dry ones like the Plantain, the Gramigna, the Horsetail, or the Cold-Humid like the Portulaca, red poppy, and lettuce.

Galen distinguishes the causes that generate liver disease and he places them in a kind of polarity; in one of the two extremes, it is the obstruction, an event which, directly or indirectly, is connected with Phlegm (Cold) and with viscous Moisture. At the other extreme is a liver disease caused by a liver that is too hot to produce bile perverse yellow.

In the first case, the Hot and Dry plants are active, which with their "assertive" virtue, they clean the ducts and so on by doing they restore normal function. In the second case the same drugs having nothing to open a stereo would increase the hepatic heat, aggravating in this case, use plants fresh, emollient, and slightly astringent. Milkweed administered the same recipe both in the case of Heat and of obstruction-Coldness with the difference that in the second a chance he paired it with wine.

Potion for icterics: Chicory juice 300ml. With the pure fever, without fever with the addition of 150 ml. Of wine According to Niceratus (Relief of Asclepias of Bithynia I century BC), yellow bile can be drained through the renal system: dried chickpeas, 300g. Rosemary leaves, fennel, marsh asparagus, of each one handful: Make the decoction in 3 liters of abundant water; yes administers such to those who have an excess of Heat; mixed with Wine to those who do not have this excess.

Another herbal recipe is Pastilla (also called Elettuario), is a paste obtained by mixing drugs pulverize with a liquid suitable (Wine, Water, Honey, Vinegar, Vegetable Juices ...) and if any formed pills (hence the term modern "tablet").

A certain degree of heat is essential to ensure that the the liver performs its functions correctly; the liver, in fact along with the heart and stomach, it is the hottest organ, however if the heat is excessive pathologies could be created, above all the inflammatory, but also gallstones, thirst, fever, irritating dermatoses; while painful syndromes they will have exacerbations.

Yellow bile will be formed to a greater extent than the other moods accentuating the pathologies described above. Blood it will increase the circulating Heat, overload the Heart and it too will become too hot so that you can have: plethora, hypertension, fever, redness.

In the renal apparatus, there will be stones, and in the apparatus genitourinary inflammation will occur.

The Spleen, which is an organ that works well with a a moderate degree of heat, it will be overheated, creating so a perverse Mood; that is, Black Bile / Melancholy it will be denser, heavier with a burning note.

The Warm liver is recognized by the "habitus" of the subject;

yellowish skin and sclera, easy irritability, violent aggression and slight asymmetry of the face, with eye contracted/displaced right and also reddened sclera an inflamed, even a so red skin generalized, especially that of the face, indicate liver overheating. As for the phenomenon of obstruction, second the Humoral Doctrine, the perfect functionality of organs are connected to the flow of moods, therefore all organs not receiving the yellow Bile bearer of Organic fire stagnate for coldness and humidity this type of affection is to be used in plants warm enough and fluidifying, which favor the the normal flow of moods.

- Hepatic deobstruent (even with mild inflammation): Leaves nettle 20%, Maidenhair 20%, Centaurea minor 5%, Absinthe 5%, Chicory 20%, Elecampane 10%, Rosemary 10%, Asparagus 10%. In the form of decoction, 20 g. a day, prepared with fluid extracts 50/100 drops per day, extracts dry 2/4 tablets a day. To make the decoction in place of the water, you can use the cooking water of the chickpeas (without salt) The de-clogging capacity is thus enhanced without however, disturb in case of possible inflammation.

Again you can use a laxative plus stronger than the previous one: Senna 30%, Eucalyptus 10%, Mint,10%, Licorice 20%, Fennel 20%, Combreto 10% (This is an example of a modernized "laxative" formula for constipated subjects with obstructed liver).

- Hepatic-Depurative and Diuretic Cooling: Burdock 20% o Chicory, 20% Capelvenere, 20% Parietaria or Rose Fruits Canina, Horsetail 15%, Gramigna 15%, Red Poppy 10%. Below form of decoction 20 g. per day, prepared with fluid extracts 50/100 drops per day, dry extracts 2/4 compressed al day.Also, once a week, administer a Laxative based on Manna or Tamarindo. Syria

- Another leading figure in traditional medicine

The Mediterranean but which at the same time represents a case in its own right is Paracelsus.

Paracelsus can be considered on the one hand traditionalist, on the other, a revolutionary.

He is conservative concerning the great truths of the Church, a fundamental principles of Astrology and Alchemy, but skeptical and rebellious, both practically and underneath the theoretical one, towards the opinions supported by various medical schools.

If Paracelsus had lived in our day, he would be without it doubt a champion of all those specialties that official medicine looks to this day with distrust (osteopathy, iridology, kinesiology ...).

Paracelsus' main interest was to find the correlations between man and the cosmos; true to conception of man as microcosm, he placed the firmament in man's body, according to his favorite theory of the Astrum in corporate. According to him, the doctor should know the wonders of nature and the singular correspondence of the human microcosm with the cosmos, not only with the visible universe but also with the Arcana Invisibles of the cosmos, with the mysteries.

Reading Paracelsus, one often comes across the mystery of Melusine. Melusina is a wonderful creature, which on the one hand, it belongs to folklore, but on the other hand, to Paracelsus' secret alchemical doctrine.

In his conception, the Melusine dwell in the blood, e since the blood is the original site soul, it can be assumed that it is a kind of Vegetative soul.

In essence, this creature is nothing more than a variant of the Spiritus Mercurialis, which in the fourteenth and the fifteenth century was depicted as a monster feminine: she is a water fairy with a fishtail or snake. In ancient French legend, it is the mother of the counts of Lusignan.

When her husband surprised her once with the tail of fish, which she had to bring only every Saturday, the day of Saturn, she was forced to return to the kingdom fair, since her secret had been discovered.

The Melusina is on the same level as the sirens and nymphs, creatures that have their home in the water.

Paracelsus Melusina appears as a variant of the the mercurial serpent, therefore with the ability to metamorphosis and gifts therapeutic.

Paracelsus, as already mentioned above, gives a lot of importance to stars, and to the symbols through which nature communicates with the man.

In the time of Paracelsus, astrology was not considered a pastime like today, but it was considered to be on par with a science, think that even Kepler he was interested in astrology. Paracelsus affirmed that: *"The Stars do not force; they only determine the basic psychic energies marking of a stronger one marks the elective impulses "*.

"The first purpose that comes true in the hour of conception demonstrates what nature will want to accomplish in future ... How the sun gives its rays, spreading its own the force from the zenith of its orbit to man, even the stars they yield to man their rays and their strength, and this not only in elementary way, like the sun that warms, or like the moon that cools, but also using sensitive forces, such as art, wisdom, skill or intelligence, which yield to man their lights, and like the sun that gives its own to the body, like the sun that pierces the glass, the constellation it passes through man with all the qualities of him and penetrates him like rain in the soil, which then bears fruit thanks to that rain, as the earth bears little fruit without the help from above, man's wisdom will be little without the stars ... Yet God did not create the planets and other stars of heaven why they commanded men and why were their masters (Paracelsus-The Treasury of treasures). Speaking of the signatures instead, he writes: "There is nothing in which nature does not have place the sign of her, so that you can recognize everything for these signs.

Like plants that grow in the form inherent in theirs nature, man too is brought into the form that corresponds to the nature of him; and like forms reveal the nature of each plant, so the signatures reveal the nature of man ... and the art of signs teaches to give to everyone the right name according to its innate qualities, so that a wolf does not it will never be said lamb, nor will it be said of a dove which is one fox ... The same happens in physiognomy, which is formed and arranged according to the content ... The architect of nature is so much skillful that does not adapt the mood to the form, but the form

that is, the form of man adapts to the species of the heart of him ".

The theory of the Signatures was mainly applied to the kingdom vegetable, hence the resemblance of a plant to an organ of the human body could suggest its use to cure disturbances.

The leaf of the Pulmonaria, for example, recalling the the shape of a lung, it was used to treat The Celandine, due to the presence of yellow-orange latex contained in its branches, was given to cure the liver and jaundice. The Bean resembles the shape of a kidney it was used for kidney ailments.

Euphrasia was used and still is used to treat eye inflammation because of the dark spot present in its corolla recalls those present in the iris.

The Walnut was used to cure the intellectual fatigue given its resemblance to the brain.

The Convovolo for its tangled and crawling appearance it appeared similar to the intestine, so it came used for intestinal colic. Mandragora for its root in the shape of a human body was considered a magical plant, capable of both maddening and bring a person back to his senses, so it was used both for mental illnesses than for the practices of magic.

The skull-like poppy capsule came used for headaches.

So it is as if nature through the language of symbols and signs would suggest its properties; the intuitive man who knows how to get in touch with nature can learn to know it.

According to Paracelsus, the stars are the models, the molds, the shapes and also the matrices of all plants.

Using the force of attraction each star generates on land a grass that corresponds to it.

According to the vegetable Spagyric, which was used by Paracelsus, when a medicinal herb is harvested, is important to take into account the moon phase and, especially if operate day or night, since with the sun you do not operate on Mercurial plants and with the Moon do not manipulate plants Sulfur.

Sulfur is the soul; it is gold not in the act but still in potency The symbol that identifies this Essential is a triangle with the vertex at the top and a cross on the baseAnd the Fire, solar and golden force, which dominates on the cross of the elements.

The Merkur or spirit is the jumble of psycho-vital energies, constituting something intermediate between the thick and the subtle, the corporeal and the incorporeal, to be the way of the vital principle of the animal or plant organism.

Bearer of cold together with water and earth; it is the center of the radical Moist, which nourishes and conserves wet and cold influences and sorts them into the body parts in which it houses.

The Merkur or passive principle is called la by philosophers "Strong force of each Force," that is, that Energy so much powerful, to overwhelm everything, but capable if addressed in the right direction, to throw open the doors of more than

It is under the sign of Water and represents all of them the aspects, both the negatives and the positives, and therefore indicates the female nature ruled by the Moon, white and milky, as white and milky are the waters acidulous, which constitute the vehicle, through which we can feel it.

The ancients called Upper Waters the whole Universe and hence the cosmic energy that permeates the whole principle the engine of all life and all movements Merkur consists of a crescent moon in horizontal, above the circle of Chaos, and below the cross.

The Sal or body is the third of the Essentials and represents the physicality or terrestrial entity, also called Saturn.

The force of the Earth acts there, which governs and determines the heaviness of "our lead," hardness and tangibility of the animal or plant body, which manifests itself through the element Calcium. Merkur, Sal, and Sulfur are three parts that makeup one body. Sal is the fixed for antonomasia or Saturn that devours its children, the Time-Chrono that corrupts and dissolves the material body.

Legend has it that Saturn-Cronus, ancient King of Olympus, he knew that one day would be dethroned by one of his sons, than to attempt to escaping his fate one by one devours all of his own his children, until his wife, Rea Silvia (Rea because she knew that that the husband was doing) feeds the husband some stones wrapped in blankets making him believe that yes it was about his children. In doing so, he manages to save one taking him to an island where the goat will suckle him Amalthea, The saved child, will become the future king Olympus, or Jupiter-Zeus who will place the goat in firmament becoming the constellation of Capricorn the myth shows both the despotic side and the generous side of sign.

Cronus is the matter, but the essence is hidden right in it. In fact, Saturn comes from Sero = to sow: in Latin vi are two verbs "Heero" of different origin, the one that means "to sow," the other "to attack."

In the Seed, Saturn attaches the essence to the substance. The Church in fact, it makes the birth of Jesus fall right under the sign of Capricorn, the birth of Christ, indeed reveals the spirit that you manifests through matter, the spirit that incarnates archaic symbols, the Zodiac is certainly among the most universal and Mythology derives its origin from astrology. In the Sal, the Gold is present but potentially waiting to be awakened by Volatile principles.

It is the black stone, "alchemy" (from Arabic) that through various passages, it becomes more and more pure and subtle until to reach a state of perfection. Some alchemists in in the past, they believed that transmutation was possible of metals, i.e., transforming lead into gold, when in reality it is a metaphor of the soul, a symbol of rough nature man but that through various tests and the knowledge and love can reach the light of spirituality, or the Golden stage of perfection.

In addition to the cross of the salts, it is taken in consider the cross of the elements, for the ancient sages in fact, the whole universe was made up of four forces or subtle elements: Fire, represented by a triangle with the vertex at the top, the Air, represented as the first but with a the horizontal line below the vertex.

Water, represented by an inverted triangle Earth, represented as Water but with a line horizontal before the vertex.

Earth, by nature, is cold. This frigidity makes the body heavier and denser, this density makes it less passable by light was created in the midst of the waters with which it is always mixed; it seems that the Creator made it arid in surface to make it suitable for the life of plants and Its sponginess makes it suitable for absorbing others elements and to cause the inner Fire, from the center to surface, may through its pores, push the virtues of elements to prepare the seeds for a generation.

These seeds thus prepared, then receive the heat life-giving heavenly, which they attract with magnetic love; then the germ develops and gives its fruit Nature, wanting the Earth to be the matrix of the mixed, the continuously warms, thanks to the heat of the celestial Fire and of the central one, and adds the humid nature of Water, for aided by the two principles of generation, the heat and the wet does not remain sterile, becoming the vessel in which you all generations complete.

This is why the Earth is said to contain others elements.

Water has an average density between that of Air and that of the Earth. It is the menstruation of Nature and the vehicle of seeds. Become volatile to escape the onslaught of Fire turning into steam.

It takes on all forms, more changeable than Proteus needs of the Earth; it also possesses a nature similar to the first material of the world, for which it easily assimilates the image.

The Chaos from which everything came was like a vapor or substance humid similar to a faint smoke.

Water, therefore, participating like Air and of Earth is positioned in the middle; lighter than Earth, more heavy of the Air, it is always mixed with the one and with the other. At the smallest rarefaction, it seems that it leaves the Earth, however take the form of Air, and then return to Earth.

The nature of Water is rather humid than cold, as it is thinner and more light-penetrable than it is there Earth Dryness is as much an effect of cold as of hot; in fact, the former condenses and dries up the humid, and this is can see in snow and ice. If winter is rigid brings dryness to the roots, hindering the humid vital, then the plants dry out. Therefore it is wrong affirm that cold is one of the qualities of water, but neither indeed, it is an enemy; in fact, both cold and heat burn them plants; cold with an astringent effect, heat with a dilating effect.

Water is the cause of revolutions, of disorder, of gods whirlwinds, the turmoil and upheaval observed in the Air and on the Earth. It disturbs the order of the seasons and nature, bringing harm and benefit in equal measure.

Air is light and not visible; it is the receptacle for all seeds.

It is an element that is always full, diaphanous, and the readiest to take on the most alien qualities, as easily

He abandons them. Philosophers call him Spirit, speaking of Great Work, as it contains the vital spirits of all bodies.

The sustenance of Fire, animals, and vegetables, as they die if they are deprived of it. Nothing would be born in the world if it were not for its penetrating force an iridescent; nothing can resist its rarefaction. The zone higher than Air, near the Moon, is pure, and it is not igneous because it is not contaminated from no vapor coming from below. The middle region of the Air collects the most subtle sulfurous influences, released by the vapors denser, which wander here and occasionally ignite, giving life to the meteor phenomenon.

In the lower region of the Air, they thicken and become they accumulate the Earth's vapors, and then fall back, for their own weight under the action of cold. Air is saturated with vapors, but these are not seen except in the form of clouds.

The ancients placed Fire in the highest region of the Air, as they considered him the most subtle and incorporeal of the The Creator has accumulated a fiery spirit in the Sun.

Principle of movement and a sweet warmth that communicates a all bodies, exciting and developing the Fire that is in it innate.

He keeps the principle of the generation of life in animals seems to have established its principal seat in the heart, which it communicates it to all parts of the body, as well as the Sun to everything the universe.

The Fire of nature favors the passage in the seeds from power to act. The Fire of nature favors the passage in the seeds from power to act.

As soon as it stops acting, every apparent movement does it stops, as well as any sign of life.

The movement has light as its principle and heat as the effect, for this the lack of light and heat produces great disasters in the bodies. The heat also penetrates most bodies hard and dense, and the hidden and inert nature animates you; while the light only penetrates diaphanous bodies, wherever, wherever it is generation, there is necessarily Fire as the cause efficient It cannot be affirmed opposition and opposition between Water and Fire, as there is no water without Fire, as they always act together in the generation in fact, there is a solid bond capable of uniting the individuals elements and higher things with the lower; in the world indeed everything is produced in harmony and union.

The ancients held that the Sun ruled so particular to Fire and the Moon to Water, as they considered the star as the source of the Fire of Nature and the Moon like the principle of the wet.

This made Hippocrates claim that the elements of the Fire and Water can do everything since they contain all.

It appears that Cardinal Rohan attempted in various ways to producing the philosopher's stone but failing in his he intent called Cagliostro, who knew to be a expert connoisseur of these things.

The latter told him to throw everything away and seek the Philosopher's stone in another way.

Be considered a directly derived practice from Alchemy. The Crusaders transmitted this to the West knowledge through the Templars.

Many famous people contributed to the spread in Europe of Alchemy: in addition to Paracelsus, Dante Alighieri, Tommaso d'Aquino, Ruggero Bacone ... Alchemy is there the science that teaches the mysterious dynamism that presides over transmutation of natural bodies The alchemist is an imitator of nature, a philosopher who seeks to through analogy realize what God the creator did in the universe, then work a divine transmutation. The alchemist divided into two Branche this science: - The Alchemy which represents it study of philosophy and the search for divine transmutation alchemical knowledge applied to the vegetable is Spagyric.

The word Spagyric is formed from the Greek "space," which means to divide and "agheiro," which means to unite.

Spagyric is the preparation of tinctures and essences taken from officinal plants through a complex procedure the first traces of a very ancient discipline can be found in fact, already among the Egyptians who considered it a practice sacred Spagyria is the synthesis of initiatory knowledge born from the relations between the Greco-Roman culture with the Arab one.

Spagyric separates the three basic principles of plants: Salt, Sulfur, Mercury, purifies them separately and brings them together in one new plant Spagyria also does not only use the principle active of the plant, but treats the plant as a set of components that work in synergy, thus recognizing the plant as a whole, composed not only of molecules but also from a "soul" that makes a plant an entity with its essence and not a simple chemical laboratory.

Simple tincture harnesses the medicinal power of the plant only partially; the spagyric preparation instead of using the the whole plant fully awakens its potential.

The Spagyric preparation is based on the alchemical concepts from which derives and makes it's own the three states of being: Salt, Mercury and Sulfur: only the alchemical preparation that contains these elements is a true Spagyric elixir and exalt all the virtues of medicinal plants. Operations to obtain the product spagyric, called the Fifth Essence, are very complex.

The three elements must first be separated through cooking and distillation.

It is extracted through steam distillation the oil, the ash is obtained from the calcination, and with the fermentation is obtained from alcohol.These extracts are then purified and finally combined in a single preparation with a a complicated procedure that also takes into account the planets of the phases of the moon. In the green alchemy during the day, yes they must separate, purify and reunify plants. At night instead, we work within ourselves in our interiority.

The healing powers of plants can be enhanced with the pronounced word and can reach the maximum effectiveness if we help its action, with the conscience the will, if the evoked powers are also used for the good of others.

Tinctures must be upgraded with the rule 7x7x7 that is with seven hours of circulation, seven of a break, seven times, or almost a week of work.

According to Chinese medicine, all organs follow a rhythm daily, alternating peak energy phases with others in which energy decreases. This belonging of the organs to hours night or day, it should apply analogously to corresponding tinctures.The kidneys, gallbladder, lungs, liver and the circulatory system belong to the lunar cycle; while stomach, heart, large intestine, bladder, spleen, and pancreas, yes place in the solar cycle.

An example of a Spagyric laboratory can be done with Juniper berries :

- They take 1 kg. We wash them and put them in soak in as much rainwater so that the berries are covered by at least two fingers, and we leave them that way for 24-36 hours.

After that time, we remove the water and throw it in how many natural and non-natural impurities are dissolved there; then we dry the berries and crush them in a mortar of stone, until they are reduced to pulp.

We take it all and put it in a flask by mouth wide, which we close hermetically and put it in a room at a temperature of about 39-40 °

for at least 14 days (modern systems such as pillows can be used electric, incubators or the ancient methods and that is the the heat of manure, best of all is the time of horse, as this animal, eats grass and oats in the seeds is hidden the Astrum or sky terrestre del mixed) prefixed, we take everything and insert it into a balloon of 6 liters, and we mount all the equipment on top of it the distillation of essential oils.

The best method is the steam current, slow but safe. After about 20 hours, they collect in the fitting where the oil is deposited, about 16 cubic centimeters (1.58%) of beautiful yellow-green color and with a concentrated smell of Juniper.

Usually, the pharmacopeia gives for 1 kg. of said plant 0.2 to 2.7% etheric substance.

The smallest parts of water contained in the oil are separated with a separating funnel.

Now what is left must be distilled again in the flask, after having poured it into a container plus suitable, i.e., with a wide neck, at a temperature suited to Nature. Such an operation takes about 4-6 days and does not have to never be interrupted; at the end, we will have the distillate and the residual mass of the berries, with some liquid.

Now you have to distill the liquid left with the plant, but yes will have to increase the temperature, as it has the sour nature, which is the real Merkur that the lyrics speak of.

The great physician Gosset who cured the Sun King wrote.

"Kabbalistic Revelations of an Extracted Universal Medicine from wine ", where we read: -" In all kingdoms, it begins with the separate the volatile part from the fixed part which in the vegetable kingdom is the Sulphurea part that rises for first, in the mineral is the acid, and in the animal the volatile Sal So in the vegetable kingdom it forms essential or the Soul of the mixed consists in the humid volatile the greasy plane and you have to purify it very well, separating it from the other principles. This etheric oil is different from the coarse, as the former is very volatile and is extracted from fermented liqueurs; the other is more fixed and will be processed in followed, to become similar to the first, with which it will be joint, to make a single substance.

- Now we have two things: Sulfur, which is "the humid volatile the unctuous plane "and the Merkur or acid spirit.

The latter must be distilled until the phlegm from the vinegar until it remains at the bottom of the balloon thick and oily silt. Vinegar must be rectified a "bain-marie," so that only the residual parts rise of phlegm; then what remains must be exposed to the air for 4-5 days, sheltered from the sun and rain, until sour taste appears.

Later it will rectify 7 times again, putting between 5 days of circulation in a bain-marie.

The vinegar obtained is called by the philosophers "Aura psychic ".Now there are

1) The residue of the berries left at the bottom of the ball.

2) The thick and oily residue, the rest of the first distillation of the acid spirit. It must be extracted from both residues, the salts. Take the berries now reduced in gruel and put in an iron pan, turn on the stove, while in the container you pour the alcohol of wine, fino to imbimb the vegetable; it waits until it remains of the brownish ash (about 60 gr.).

The same thing is done with residue number 2, and it is obtained about 30 gr. of brownish-black ash.

We have two ashes, and we must extract their respective salts.

We take the first ash and put it in the capsule extraction, while in the flask in contact with the fire, we put 500 gr. of distilled water (i.e., without salts) all and after about 5 hours, which correspond to 12 ascents capsule emptyings (i.e., three emptyings for each of the four elements) the salts were extracted from the ash are dissolved in distilled water.

The whole has a yellow-orange-dark color, as the liquid is saturated to the maximum, and we distill it until you see the crystals of a whitish Sal. 100 gr. of water distilled, the salts are dissolved, and the liquid evaporated; this we repeat it 7 times, and we will obtain, from 60 gr. of ash, 7 gr.

Of Sal of the salts, white as snow. This 7 gr. Of Sal in a crucible, cover with the lid, and insert in an oven, capable of at least 600 ° temperature. After 8 hours please turn off the oven and let it cool for at least 24 hours, then the crucible is removed, uncovered, and we will see attached to the bottom, a white molten mass.

It is dissolved with boiling distilled water, evaporated and we will have our 7 gr. of Sal of salts, at a truly excellent degree of purity. With the second ash, we will do the same thing, and there we will find, from 30 g. of ash, 4.5 of Sal of the salt of Sulfur Now we have:

1) The Sulfur (essential oil-spiritetheric)

2) The Merkur

3) The Sal (the Sal of the salts, which is the fixed body and the Sal of the salt of Sulfur, volatile).

We have to get the yellow oil, the black oil, the oils below (the essential oil is an oil from above), and the Sal del Merkur.

We still take 300 g. of Juniper roots, crush them in a mortar, and put them in a very resistant flask of approx 4 liters. The entire equipment for the oils of under.

The aforementioned balloon must be placed on a tripod, in inclined position, taking care to place it on a net insulator to prevent the tripod metal from twisting to the heat.

The balloon must be connected to a normalized tube, of length of one meter, and at the other end take a another 2-liter flask via a Y-fitting 2-liter container must be contained in a saucepan large enough to put water and ice.

A Liebig cooler is inserted along with a meter and a half to which a vase is inserted at the end of the tube of expansion and a bubbler half full of vinegar;

The two last containers are traps to capture the oils The inclined balloon with the roots must be caged with baking foil so that the the temperature at least 600 °, otherwise the yellow oils blacks, hidden in the depths of the plant.

When that caloric content has been reached, in the tube that goes down to the flask contained in the pot, yes he will see a thick vapor filling him, followed by a trickle oily yellow, which will begin to pour into the container a little bit, the black oil will go down, and after 4-5 hours, nothing will come out with charred roots. Leave to cool for a while day and then the various pieces are taken apart.

They take the two oils now mixed and put in a funnel separator, which will hang in a perch from laboratory, securing it with rubber-coated pliers it will leave in this position for a few hours, to separate the water from the oil completely; then the cap of the small tap for pouring the oily liquid. When it is about to pass, the water will close the exit.

I about 80 g. of oil will be placed in a 500 g balloon. Is let yourself be slowly distilled in a bain-marie, being careful that the heat is not too exuberant.

After about a week, we will have 70 g. of very refined oil and degreased, ready to be combined with the essential one. With the coal left in the flask, the usual salt extraction will be done which we will add to the Sal de Salts.

The sorrel or Merkur we have must be redistilled for at least three times, and the residue will be made concentrate until the consistency of baby food. From this, with the appropriate operations you will get the Sal del Merkur.

We need to combine the three salts: the sal of salts + the ps del Merkur + the Sal del Sulfur, putting them in heated vinegar and stir everything with a glass rod, until complete dissolution, let it cool down, and you will pour the oils; let everything settle, then shake well well and let's distill very slowly, all the time it takes (about a week).

At the bottom, only a light veil should remain oily, with some trace of Sal crystals and the distillate should have a sweet Juniper smell; the taste slightly sour and bitter, but with a sweet residual taste.

The common Juniper is Juniperus communis, the most widespread in world, while there is another plant, the Juniperus oxycedrus, typical of the Mediterranean basin, from which red fruits are extracts an acrid and caustic oil that was once used by Romans to embalm the dead is still used today in dermatology to manufacture numerous ointments.

There is also a third type of Juniper, Juniperus sabina, the whose oil was used as an emmenagogue and abortion.

Juniper wood was considered unassailable by woodworms, while the burnt rind is reduced to ashes a mixed with water, it was used for leprosy and mange; moreover, in 1870 in the hospitals of Paris, it was eradicated a smallpox epidemic thanks to juniper fumigation this ability to keep Juniper away from diseases it was also used to ward off evil spirits while the smoke obtained from the burnt Juniper was seen as a symbol of ascension towards Christ.

The Juniper infusion serves to expel the lactic acid that it is formed after physical exertion.

The green leaf extract has a repellent action energetic towards insects and is also an antidote against their poison.

The fresh fruit exerts a bronchodilating action, therefore useful in the chronic affections of smokers.

Promotes the healing of ulcerated wounds; distilled in steam current provides beneficial water for the aching joints. In the 2nd century BC a Juniper berry-based diuretic wine to combat the Fenella, stones, and inflammations of the passages urinary. Today it is used in cooking to flavor the game, while from the herbalist tradition it is kept its use for urinary infections and pains articular.

In the alchemical texts of the Middle Ages, the tree appears frequently and generally represents the growth of arcane substance and its transformation into Gold philosophical Zosimus (2nd century AD alchemist) I would have said that the transformation process is like a a tree well cared for and sprayed and that in contact with hot air humid, it bears fruit and blossoms. The Whole is also found in the most a small particle of matter, like a miniature or a hologram, therefore the Macrocosm is in the Microcosm, in everything animate and inanimate, so every grain becomes wheat and every metal becomes gold, and the little man becomes great man, in fact, the moral equivalent of physical transmutation into gold is self-knowledge.

The alchemists' tree is the solar tree, bearer of fruit, and the lunar tree with silver fruits, masculine and feminine symbols. Also, in alchemy, there is the tree of gods seven planets symbolizing the seven stages of the process Each part of the tree is connected to a planet:

Saturn, Mars, Jupiter, and Venus form the trunk, while the Sun and Luna contains the seeds. The tree of seven planets is metallic earth, and the trunk is red mixed with black. Its leaves are similar to marjoram and are thirty, as the days of a lunar cycle. Its flower is yellow, while the soil in which it is sown consists of Mercury purified.

Another alchemical meaning of the tree is the cut tree:

An ancient Egyptian fairy tale tells that the hero Bata laid his soul in the tallest flower of an Acacia, when the tree comes knocked down, it is found in the form of a seed, like this Bata, who had been killed, came back to life. When he was killed for the second time in the form of a bull, from his blood two trees were born, when these two were felled a splinter from the trunk fertilized the queen, who she brought into the world a son who became pharaoh; Bata was reborn to become one sacred person. In this story, the tree is a symbol of transformation and reincarnation of the soul that through various experiences, it reaches more and more states evolved, as well as in the alchemical process we start from raw material until it reaches the most precious metal 13th-century Arab alchemist describes a tree with four types of flowers of different colors: four is the number of the earth.

The Book of Enoch (hermetic text) of the second century BC speaks of a tree whose fruits will be the food of the elect, the tree is compared to the Vine, in the Middle Ages, the philosophical tree was called Vitis.

The miraculous tree or plant is located in the mountains; correlation between tree and mountain is not accidental in fact, both are instruments of the celestial journey of the shaman.

As the seat of the transformation, the tree assumes a feminine and maternal meaning in the representations Hellenistic Isis has the appearance of a Melusina, and her symbols I am the torch, the Vine, and the palm tree.

A Greek legend tells that when the Vine did not have one more name, she used to climb other trees, forming a vegetable forest from which she gushed the red juice of hers fruits.

At the sight of the red bunches, the child Bacchus remembered the oracles of the fateful Rea, his nurse of him, and decided to derive the wine from those fruits. Rea's presence in the background of this myth alludes to the Great Cretan Goddess who ruled over plants and animals, accompanied or adorned with various attributes, by the lion, to the bull, to the snakes.

From the cult of the Great Mother, the god of wine emerged in Crete, of bulls and women, or Bacchus / Dionysus, a symbol of liberation from bonds through a state of ecstasy that is been described by Nietzsche: "Under the Dionysian spell not only does the bond between man and man shrink, but it also estranged nature celebrates its festival again reconciliation with his lost son, man.

The earth spontaneously offers her gifts and the wild animals rocky and desert lands approach peacefully. Now the slave is a free man, now they break all the rigid, hostile boundaries that necessity, will or the brash fashion has been established among men.

Now in the gospel of universal harmony, everyone feels not only reunited, reconciled, fused with his neighbor, but even one with it, as if Maia's veil had been torn and now waving in shreds in front of the mysterious original unity.

By singing and dancing, man manifests himself as a member of a higher community: he has unlearned to speak and to walking and is on the point of flying into the sky dancing ".

The Sumerians also knew a goddess known as Goddess Vite or Mother vine, the vine was in fact called "grass of life," while Christ took the Vine as a symbol of him, stating: "I am the real vine ".

Inspired by the ancient tradition, both Greek and Jewish-Christian, the Renaissance ones elaborated allegories where the Vine, with the fermented juice of her fruit, could be a symbol of happiness or a symbol of relief and help towards the needy.

Joy was represented by a young woman supported to an elm surrounded by vines; the allegory of help towards the needy, it is instead represented by a man dressed in white with a purple cloak, his head is surrounded by a wreath of olive trees and is illuminated by celestial rays, while around his neck she wears a necklace with a heart-shaped pendant.

The white of the robe represents the purity of mind and the sincere desire and without ulterior motives to help others, the purple cloak equally represents Charity, rays that descend from heaven allude to divine help, the head of man is surrounded by an olive wreath representing the peace and mercy. Man has his right arm outstretched to mean that any help requires strength (the arm right, as well as the whole right part of the body, are connected to action as dominated by the rational hemisphere). The left arm instead grabs a pole driven into the ground sinuously surrounded by a vine while a stork him stands beside. The stork is the emblem of filial piety for the loving care that he knows how to give to his children, while the stake he supports the vine represents the support that one must know how to offer to others.

The Philosophical Tree is also represented as Oak is like myrtle. In ancient Greece, the names of many heroines or amazons had the same root as myrtle:

Myrtò, Myrìne ... Myrtò was an Amazon who fought together with other companions of her, the Attic hero Theseus. Myrsìne instead, she is remembered for her warrior courage aroused the jealousy of young people who, for this reason, the killed, later she was transformed into

Myrtle, The combination of Myrtle with Amazons, underlines both the close link between the plant and femininity, that the strangeness to the Greek Indo-European tradition.

The plant was associated with Venus / Aphrodite and the Etruscan goddess Turan The legend told about Herostratus tells that his ship near the Egyptian coast was surprised by one terrible storm, then Aphrodite intervened to help him and yes she manifested by giving birth to myrtle leaves on the statuette of the goddess that Herostratus carried with him.

The miracle reassured the sailors and increased their vigor allowing them to reach the shore safe and sound.

Indeed, Myrtle has energetic and invigorating qualities.

Myrtle was used to crowning the bride and groom during the wedding banquet as a symbol of fertility, also in Rome it was planted in public places because Venus didn't she oversaw only marital unions but also a those policies offering her beneficial energy peace. In fact, on the republican coins a a sprig of Myrtle together with Concordia.

The plant also symbolized the victory obtained without bloodshed in military campaigns.

But Myrtle was also considered a plant In ancient Greece, it was said that Dionysus descended into Hades.

To free his mother, Semele killed by a thunderbolt of Zeus had had to leave a Myrtle plant in exchange.

Like Dionysus, he is at the same time god of light and god of gods underworld, killed and resurrected, the Myrtle at the same time has both one the luminous and auspicious value that a funeral and a hellish one like all plants associated with the Great Mothers.

From a botanical point of view, Myrtle belongs to the family of the blueberries to which also the Eucalyptus, the Tree belongs tea and cloves ... all plants that do not grow in the Mediterranean basin, Myrtle is, in fact, the only one a representative of the family growing up on the coast Mediterranean Berries are used in Sardinia for aromatize a well-known liqueur, but you can also get one vinous tincture with digestive properties.In the Middle Ages date the its association with Venus, goddess of love, was advised as an aphrodisiac to pulverize the leaves and sprinkle them on the whole body.

In the 17th century, from the distillation of leaves and flowers, a refreshing and invigorating cosmetic, still known called Acqua Degli Angeli. In the Mediterranean tradition, the uses the main ones are basically the same as today: yes in fact, recognized the Mirto, and still recognize themselves today, thanks to toxic, anti-inflammatory, and balsamic properties With the oil contained in the leaves, the Blueberry.

A syrup can be prepared with Myrtle leaves expectorant: put 75 g. of myrtle leaves in water boiling.

Leave to rest for 6 hours, filter, and add 1 kg. and 750 g. of sugar.Mix well and put everything back on fire, causing it to thicken.Doses: 2-4 tablespoons a day.

Chapter 6

The Medieval Botanical Garden-

Now I would like to talk about a botanical garden attached to an ancient Benedictine abbey located in Perugia, where in addition to many plants of herbal interest are found also many medieval symbols and allegories.

Inside the garden, a journey takes place through the symbols and myths that lead to re-reading Creation is key spiritual, if not animistic, according to the typical view of medieval man.

In this symbolic garden, there is no scan chronological of events, time plays a role relative, symbolisms, arcane languages and cryptic, the harmonies of numbers, the hidden virtues of plants. In the Middle Ages, the tree is identified with a man in his rush towards the sky.

Astral plants linked to signs also appear in the garden zodiacal, the herbs from which medicines are obtained simple, as well as the herbs, used to flavor food.

The Paradise of Eden (for man medieval entrance to the monastery mimicked the entrance to earthly paradise): the specially chosen plants, the figures deliberately drawn in circular shapes, ellipticals, squares ... the measures and numbers that are anything but random have a strong symbolic meaning.

On the one hand, the wood represents the "dark forest," a place menacing and full of shadows, on the other hand, a sacred place, from living in solitude and asceticism. The medieval garden, and that monastic in particular arose from the man's need for time to find a more natural dimension and closer to the divine, that's why it was enriched with symbolic motifs and meanings sacred; in the Middle Ages, in fact, the vision of the world was expressed in strongly representative key; shapes, lines, numbers they take on much deeper and more hidden values than those apparent, and can be grasped by giving space to intuition and to unconscious images more than logic.

The men of the Middle Ages read nature is key animistic in fact, the management of the gardens and nature in generally, they were linked to religious practices before Christianity.

In Rome as well as in Greece, there were numerous divinities propitious to agriculture and crops.

Pan was the protector of the countryside, hunters, and especially the shepherds, while Pomona supervised the gardens and fruit trees. Priapus was another god of the fields and flocks.

Demeter / Ceres identified with the same generating force of nature, and therefore she was considered the goddess of all plants: in the honor of her in Greece, the Eleusinian Mysteries were celebrated, while a Rome celebrated the Cereralia, which lasted from 12 to 19 April, during which we ate only in the evening and yes they scattered flowers and nuts in the street.

Flora, the wife of Zephyr, was the goddess of flowers and spring, in the Floralia was celebrated in honor of her, from April 28 to 3 May If Marìca was a nymph of vegetation in general, the Meliache or Meliadi was the ash trees.

The Palila, from Pale (protector of shepherds and flocks), were rural festivals celebrated on April 21 during which the peasants purified the stables and sheepfolds. The Suovetaurilia in honor of Mars instead consisted in the sacrifice of a pig, of one sheep or a bull, to purify the fields after a battle.

Vertumnus, the divinity of gardens and gods, played a particular role gardens, but which presided over the change of seasons thanks to of his ability to the transformer; in fact, in love with Pomona he used this talent to conquer her; so yes he transformed once into a plowman, another reaper, a winemaker and even in an older woman, four characters symbolizing the four seasons, when he showed himself in his royal guise he appeared covered with fruit from head to toe, as well as the painter Arcimboldo represented him.

The journey inside the symbolic garden is faced with it spirit of those who want to know the religious and cultural past Western man, through the botanical symbolisms that they are in his history or moving from plant elements typical of his everyday world ten stages follow with a meaning chosen on the basis of the historical and religious consequentiality of the time.

The Primordial State - It is the first stage. There are many reminders biblical on the origin of Man.

The purity of the lines and the brightness dominate symbolizing the perfection of creation.

The Guilt - During this phase, the man knows the sin that is symbolized by the forest, dark and fraught with danger, in which Man must fight for survival; he is the symbol of the primitive earth condition and loss of innocence, it is the kingdom of darkness, where it is seen however even some flash of light, which seeps through the trees.

Rationality - In this phase, the human being learns a discerning the herbs and starting to cultivate the fields is the phase of atonement (you will work the earth with the sweat of your brow) but at the same time of the redemption from a primitive state of ugliness. Domination - Man at this stage has learned a taming nature, which is expressed by a site high panoramic view where the gaze overlooks the landscape that it appears totally dominated by Man.

Creativity - The concept of Homo dominates you Faber, the Man who sows, collects, hunts, fishes production phase.

The community - Expresses the need to live in society therefore to apply rules and laws to facilitate the coexistence between human beings.

Religiosity - Represents spiritual growth, where cloisters are reconstructions of the lost Paradise and the columns and capitals represent the momentum towards the sky.

Culture - It is the state of the Homo magister, the Man who he teaches his children and passes on his own knowledge.

Aesthetics - Man through architectural beauty expresses his thirst for the Absolute and Purity.

Holiness - The examples of the saints in the cloister follow pressing, repeated, up to the church, center and the apex of the sacredness of the site.

Medieval cathedrals were built respecting the orientation of the cardinal points: the church of the Maddalena in Vezelay is oriented so that a noon of the summer solstice, (it was believed that fell on June 24), the sun's rays fell right at center of the floor in the nave, as if constituted a kind of "path of light."

Also, the energy was taken into account magnetic, cosmic, and telluric of the land to build the church so that it was able to give off energy beneficial.

The Logo expresses the founding mentality and philosophy of Garden of the Spirit is the emblem of the most symbolic Garden then the real one: It is made up of three elements the animals, the frame, and the tree. The frame is a the arch that follows that of a medieval door dominates the scene. It is an ideal tree, a hybrid between an olive tree, a symbol of peace, a laurel, a symbol of glory and a Lives, a symbol of salvation - In Delphi, they were celebrated every eight years the Pythian Games, which took their name from the snake python, guardian of the oracle of Daphne and subjugated by Apollo: a crown of Laurel.

During the Roman Empire, the Laurel was reserved for emperors, after the prodigy narrated by Pliny in the "History natural ":" Livia

Drusilla, when she was still engaged with Cesare Augusto, one day, she saw herself fall into her lap a hen dropped by a flying eagle, unharmed, that she was holding a sprig of Laurel with her beak they advised to keep the hen and to plant the sprig near the banks of the Tiber, a place named for this reason Ad Gallinas, where shortly after a grove.

From that moment on when Caesar Augustus he celebrated his triumphs; he used to carry a sprig on his head Laurel from the grove and later became a custom common to all emperors ".

Returning to the symbolic meaning of the Logo, we note that the Tree is One, which symbolizes the principle, origin of all plant beings; There are five directions towards which it expands, in high and with two branches on each side, a symbol of Man, above is the head and laterally two arms and two legs.

Two lions are placed around the tree, one on each side, then there are three elements on each side, plus the top of the tree, so there are seven elements in all, many how many planets were known at that time?

The number five is found both in the number of ramifications, which in the leaves.

Five is the number of Man, just as it is a number creative and feminine par excellence. The low branches carry every eight leaves (Number of the Infinite), while each single branching of each branch consists of three leaves (The Three is a symbol of perfection: Sal, Merkur, Sulfur or Body, Mind, and Spirit that together create.

The tree in total has twenty-seven leaves, or three raised to the third, which amplifies the meaning inherent in the number three. The lateral branches coming from the central branch they are the ones that produce the fruits, not only in the sense material but also spiritual. The Clusters are four consisting of three fruits, four by three makes twelve that represents an emblematic and significant number stem in the upper part is straight, while in the lower part, it is a spiral, which is a symbol of infinity and movement ascensional but also a symbol of the coiled snake around the Tree of Knowledge.

The two Lions represent the animal side of Man, the struggle for survival, but it is also a symbol of courage.

In the Old Testament, the Lion had a negative value, while later assumed a positive meaning many Romanesque churches, the Lions keep watching, therefore they act as custodians of what is sacred and are often the symbol of the saints, for example, San Marco and San Girolamo the motto at the bottom of the frame, *"Virentium Virtutes,"* resumes precisely the concept of the nutritional and healthy strength of the gods.

A suffused religious symbolism animates the Logo in its.

The Tree is a cross that buds and bears fruit; it is a the meeting point between natural religiosity and Christian religiosity.

But also the memory of the Myth: Cybele, the Great Mother identifiable with the same generating force of Nature, it is here transformed into a Primordial Plant, a Great Mother Plant.

As for the colors, the Lions and the Plant are colored yellow, the color of the Sun and energy, which painted on glass in so that it has the sky as background, that is blue, become green; in fact, the yellow and the blue overlapping give like the final result is the green color, which in plants is the acquisition functional and constitutional due to the presence of chlorophyll, and which effects have a cascading impact on animals for the dependence of these on those symbolizes energy nutritional, it represents life itself.

Hildegard of Bingen had sensed that vigor and vitality that the plants appeared to possess; it was nothing but fruit of the ability to capture and emanate energy, the therefore, a plant was only an admirable synthesis.

In 1842, that is, seven centuries later, this intuition was confirmed by the discovery of the molecule of chlorophyll by Julius Meyer.

The Garden begins with Earthly Paradise when it begins the history of humanity.

You enter the Garden of Eden through a flower bed rotunda, in the center of which there is a large tree evergreen: the circular space around the plant represents the world in embryo, the visitor comes to being in a space-time dimension where it already is born the Idea (the Point, the origin of everything).

The circle is the theoretical extension of the OneCenter, of the Origin, of the primordial Point, of the One the progenitor of all numbers, the beginning of all things.

From the Center or Origin, the Whole was born, Life was born, it was born the Tree, the Tree of Life, or Cosmic Tree, was born.

The circle around the Tree is not closed, and this is a sign adaptation to the evolutionary dynamism of World.

The primeval Tree threw a bridge between the earth and the sky, between the natural and the supernatural world, between Man and God.

The Tree was the source of Life, Heat, Light, gave shape to primordial living matter vitalized the world inanimate, he procreated. The Tree stretched its feet into the earth and stretched out his arms towards the sky, support of this and the anchor of that.

The Tree lit up with the sunlight, the solar fire it attracted the vital bud higher and higher, the Tree green harnessed its energy and, in turn, was a source of energy: green was life, and the tree was nourishment.

The vertical axis of the world, the Tree was a symbol ascensional, which on one side supports the celestial sphere, the hair, and on the other, it is anchored to the earth, to the human condition by the roots.

The tree fulfilled the dream of verticalization, more than how many men or animals could have done.

It was a symbol of accelerated upward growth, a mystery of infinite regeneration, a symbol of victory over death winter, each year higher and higher and higher vital, with new shoots, new leaves, new flowers, new fruits, a symbol of life that is renewed indefinitely.

Even bare, it preserves the memory of the original perfection of the principle through the conical-curvilinear forms linked to transcendence. A symbolic and representative microcosm of macrocosm, underground or underworld, earthly or human, and aerial or celestial/divine. The species in the Garden assumes the Cosmic Tree role is the Magnolia (, Magnolia grandiflora).

Magnolias are very ancient species, certainly among the most ancient higher plants appeared on earth, as has the discovery of fossil finds dating back to Cretaceous (almost 100 million years ago).

At that time, they lived on a vast territory part of the Angiosperms, from which the most of the higher plants living today.In language of flowers, Magnolia is a symbol of whiteness due to its great white flowers.

40 meters from the Cosmic Tree is the Tree of Revelation or of Good and Evil: "Then the Lord God he planted a garden in Eden to the east and placed the man there that he had fashioned; the Lord God caused it to sprout from land all sorts of trees, attractive to the eye and good from eat ... including the tree of life in the plus part garden, along with the tree of knowledge of good and evil ... "(Genesis 2: 8-9).

The number forty is strongly symbolic because expresses the atonement; in fact, 40 were the days that Christ spent in the desert; instead, Moses spent 40 days on the Mount Sinai in Egypt to receive the tables of the law. 40 instead, it is the time span between the Resurrection and the Ascension, placed before and after Easter, the feast of Christianity symbolically represent a kind of round trip, that is, of Atonement and Redemption.

If the Cosmic Tree represents the Divine, the Tree of Good and Evil represents the human condition; in fact, if the former is large and luxuriant, the second is smaller and more fragile trees are found at the poles of an ellipse; this figure as well maintaining the original creative imprint of circularity it no longer has the absolute perfection of the circle; it is a circle deformed, which has lost its homogeneity in the three directions of the space seems to presage and anticipate the imperfect reality of what's this.

The oval shape is reminiscent of the egg, which symbolizes reality in becoming, from the point of view of sacred allegory, simulates one almond, a symbol of divine nature. The forty meters that make up the driveway they cross from one end to the other the world-ellipse passes two rivers, one coming from right and one from left, representing the Phison and the Gihon two of the four rivers that flowed out in Genesis from Eden (the other two, the Tigris and the Euphrates, are in the part opposite).

After passing the two streams, you enter more space interior, enclosed between the four rivers.

The terrestrial paradise practically consists of two ellipses concentric, an external one that has the two foci in the Tree Cosmic and in the Tree of Revelation, and an internal one enclosed between the four rivers that come out of Paradise itself Terrestrial.

In the middle of the longitudinal axis of the Garden, there is a the third tree, placed right at the center equidistant from the two trees.

To the dualistic reading of the Old Testament, it is added the central Tree representing the Tree of Light.

In Eden, therefore, an arboreal trilogy is created, which given the medieval man symbolizes the Paradise Found, a concept clearly consequent to the New Testament.

The Cosmogonic Egg placed at the center of the Earthly Paradise is divided into twelve segments, that is, twelve flower beds. Twelve are several high symbolic values: four repeated three times or three repeated four times. Four is the number symbolizing the Earth, while three is the number divine par excellence.

12 also has a high alchemical value deriving from four and from three: the multiplication of the four vital elements (earth, air, water, fire) for the three mineral elements (sulfur, salt, mercury) originates the secret of the substance of all things. Among the many meanings that could be attributed to the twelve flower beds, it was chosen, certainly not by chance, that of Zodiac; each sector corresponds in fact to a zodiac sign.

Chapter 7

Herbs and zodiac

The Zodiac, in fact, far from having a profane meaning, in Middle Ages symbolized Christ's dominion over Time and over Space. In the garden, inside each zodiacal square, they are placed some plants, in analogy with the sign, based analogies on appearance, shape, therapeutic function, flavor, color.

Aries: Rosemary, Verbena, Laurel, Narcissus, Erica, Chamomile Roman, Artichoke, Tulip, Periwinkle, Borage.

Taurus: Myrtle, Lilac, Elderberry, Strawberry wild, poppy, tarragon, safflower, rose, sage.

Gemini:

Lily of the valley, Serpillo, Celandine, Celandine, Pimpinella, Horse chestnut, Giglio, Digitalis, Savory,

Olive, Lettuce.

Cancer: Acacia, Cyclamen, Geranium, Peach, Honeysuckle, Lettuce, Walnut, Glicense, Mint, Rue, Linden, Juniper,

Caper, Thyme, Chicory, Helichrysum, Tulip, Rose.

Lion:

Geranium, Peach, Mimosa, Speronella, Saffron, Vetch, Hypericum, Borage, Gentian, Carnation.

Virgin:

Gladiolus, Wheat, Licorice, Rose, Belladonna, Bramble, Hydrangea, Apple trees, Rue, Linen, Savory, Calendula.

Weight scale:

Ivy, Lily of the Valley, Mallow, Celery, Watercress, Saffron, Hawthorn, Galega, Astro, Galega, Rosa, Ginepro.

Scorpio:

Basil, Oregano, Willow, Sage, Pine, Yew, Cumin, Oak, Soy, Cyclamen, Rosa Canina.

Sagittarius:

Primrose, Violet, Fern, Lavender, Chestnut, Chamomile, Pear, chrysanthemum, broom.

Capricorn:

Echinacea, Calicanto, Cherry, Holly, Mistletoe, Coriander, Jasmine yellow, Anise, Cypress, Laurel, Erica.

Aquarium:

Water lily, Oleander, Wallflower, Mint, Carnation, Hop, Laurel, Alchechengi, Violet, Snapdragon, Daisy, Sunflower, Coltsfoot, Nettle.

Fish: Spruce, Violet ponderosa, Watercress, Mint, Hydrangea, Jasmine, Anise, Melissa, Tarassaco, geranium.

Plants also have astral correspondences with planets: the Sanguinaria is a Solar plant, the Waterlily is the Iris are Lunar plants; the Cinquefoglie is associated with Mercury, Verbena as well as Myrtle are associated with Venus, Acanthus to Mars, Willow to Saturn, the henbane to Jupiter.

The longitudinal driveway is cut orthogonally from another a cross driveway that symbolically starting from the the monastery, place of prayer and meditation interior ideally unites the monastery to the rest of the world: one sort of symbolic testimony of the ascetic activity of monk on the one hand and social commitment on the other.

The two axes crossing orthogonally from a cross right in the center of the earthly Paradise.

All the lines, all the paths of the Earthly Paradise converge in a central point.

This central point in some configuration structures geometric is no longer curvilinear but polygonal (octagon, triangle, square), symbols of rationality

On the ground, there is a square made up of four meters per side.

As we have already said, Four is the number of the earth, more closely linked to the concrete concerning the circle.

There are four geographical directions; four were the rivers of Eden, four plants representative of the abundance of Earthly Paradise (Olivo, Melo, Vite, Fico), four evangelists (Matteo, Luca, Marco, Giovanni), four are their symbols represented in the (Calf, Aquila, Lion, Angel) ...

The sides of the square face the four quadrants of the ellipse (earth, fire, air, water) and symbolize the four senses of humor (black bile, yellow bile, phlegm, blood) from which derive the four qualities (cold, dry, wet, hot) and the four humoral complexions (melancholic, choleric, phlegmatic, sanguine).

In the square on the ground, an octagon is inscribed, which is raised concerning the whole plan of the earthly paradise.

The raised octagon represents the ascent, the mountain, the thrust towards the sky. he top of the mountain was the highest earthly elevation allowed to the man of the Middle Ages.

Four springs gush from the mountain, from which the four liquid elements that have nourished humanity: water, milk, wine, honey.

To remain in the medieval context and give the right emphasis to quality of these four elements according to the criteria of medicine of the time I report some aphorisms, as reported in Flos Medicine:

Fons aquae - Water must flow as transparent as air clear, pleasant light and fresh, and flowing fine, very pure without deposit.

And be tasteless and odorless.

Fons Lactis - Healthy is goat's milk, after that of camel, and this after that of the mare, and after that donkey: among these, the donkey gives more nourishment, but most nutritious of all are those of cow and of sheep.

Fons Mellis - The best honey is spring honey, which is sweet and thick, and shines like gold: better is what decant on the bottom.

Fons wines or drink to preserve health -

After the wine comes loquacity, after the rain the grass, knowledge after study, many after idleness things vanish; the flower is followed by the fruit, the pleasures by mourning.

The best wine generates better moods: if drinking wine in the evening made you bad, drink some early in the morning, and you will recover!

The Salerno medical school, which originated on bases religious, then had a secular development.

He dictated fundamental criteria of therapy, hygiene, and nutrition, which a great many doctors have adhered to for centuries.

The Salerno medical school had its maximum development during the twelfth and thirteenth centuries, but had previously had a strong cultural influence throughout Europe. It was a point of the encounter between the classical culture, maintained in the monasteries, and Arab science (which in turn was permeated with the ancient Middle Eastern cultures, ad example, the shutter).

The birth of the Salernitana Medical School is strictly linked to the heyday of the history of Salerno is the 10th century. The city is at the center of intense exchanges, which ones will be decisive in influencing the training of European civilization. The Mediterranean has influenced the culture, society, and the institutions of the peoples who live on its shores. At its origin, there is the fusion of culture Hebrew, Arabic, Greek, and Latin.

In addition to the teachings of Hippocrates and Galen, Constantine the African should be remembered who was an illustrious physician and philosopher at the school of Salerno, and Avicenna The first having traveled farlargo; he managed to operate a certain opening towards the new knowledge of Arab medicine.

As for Avicenna, he managed to influence the Western medicine, through the "Canon," work divided into five books: the first deals with theoretical medicine, the second of simple medicines, the third of the diseases treated a depending on their localization, the fourth of the diseases general, the fifth of the prepares = of medicinal products.

At the center of the Earthly Paradise, on the symbolic mountain, in dominant position over everything, therefore a tree grows.

Only the Tree is allowed to grow well beyond the Earth's surface: the tree, with its own strength, can grow, he can ascend far more than man and gods animals (obviously excluding birds).

With its verticality, the tree can detach itself from the earth, soar in the air, rise to the sky.

The Tree on the mountain is the Tree of Light and symbolizes the Paradise Found. It is the lamp of the world, the beacon that guides man and man clears the way.

The attribution of the Tree of Light to a centenary olive tree confirms the symbolic meaning always attributed to this splendid plant, which an ancient medieval tradition wants to grow up on the grave of Adam, the first of men.

The Tree of Light represents Christ on the cross. On the Tree of Light, both the rays converge flowerbeds of the Zodiac that the crosses' arms.

The genus Olea includes about thirty species, of which the most interesting is undoubtedly the domestic olive tree (Olea European), typical plant representative of the area Mediterranea has always occupied a prominent place in civilizations of the Mediterranean basin and neighboring ones like that Mohammed, in fact, dreamed of ascending to heaven himself along the branches of olive trees.

For Christians, the olive tree is the symbol of peace; in fact, the dove of Noah returned to the ark with an olive branch in its beak, a sign of the reconciliation of God with humanity, according to a Greek myth it was Athena / Minerva who first planted a Olive tree on Greek soil One day, the Goddess clashed with Poseidon / Neptune for possession of Attica.The first king of those lands, Cecrops, promised victory to those who created something extraordinary.Poseidon hit the ground with the trident caused a spring of salty water to gush out Athena to secure victory by giving birth to the first Olivo From that day, the Olivo was consecrated to Athena and was considered a symbol of chastity.

A campaign of Olives, from the smallest ones in Andalusia to giants of Puglia or Greece is the triumph of Light: a light not blinding, but cheerful, quiet, pacifying. A kind like the olive tree could not fail to play an important role in Traditional Mediterranean Medicine.

Leaves in decoction beyond to be used for the treatment of inflammations throat, bladder, and intestines were used especially for the treatment of infected wounds and fevers intermittent, according to an ancient tradition dating back to Roman times. In fact, before China, there were fevers cured with potions based on olive leaves and remained use until the end of the nineteenth century to replace quinine in the treatment of malaria.

One has been isolated for some decades, substance, and oleuropeoside, which acts on smooth muscle distension. The leaves are then used for activity vasodilator, hypotensive, and spasmolytic.

If the Cosmic Tree is a Magnolia and the Tree of Light a Olive, the Tree of Good and Evil, is represented by a Fig: an inconspicuous looking tree but endowed with succulent and inviting fruits that led Eva to al original sin.

The fruits of the Fig tree are called Sycons that look botanically speaking, they are false fruits, almost forming on purpose to lure those who collect them. The false fruit called precisely Siconius is formed by abnormal growth of the inflorescent receptacle, which is balloon-shaped elongated like a kind of pear.

A small hole at the apex, on the opposite side of the petiole allows the entry of a small pollinating insect the flowers contained therein. After fertilization, the fruit it becomes pulpy and sugary to attract birds who ingest the fruit-seeds which, being indigestible, come dispersed in the environment.

So the Fig tree uses the unwitting birds for disseminate.

In truth, the biblical text does not refer to fruit in particular, more generically, it is called Pomo.

The premium can be translated as Apple, but also fruit in general, in fact, "pomerium" is the orchard.

The Christian tradition has indeed identified the fruit of sin with the apple, as if the apple tree were common species in Middle East Instead, the place of origin of the Apple tree is the North Europe, although botanists have identified three other types of Apple trees from the Caucasus area regardless of the type of fruit is the symbolism of disobedience of Adam and Eve what matters.

The allegorical feature that has caused the fig to be associated with Eve is the fact that the fruits of her secrete a whitish liquid and milky similar to milk; in fact, the ancient Romans they called the plant Ficus ruminates (Ruma = breast). Metaphorically, therefore, Fig is the female plant for excellence as a galactogenic plant.

In many Italian localities, the custom of to call the pseudofrutti del Fico with the term of fig mamma or fig mammon, both evoking the concept of maternity.

However, if you trust the naturosophical theories, the maleficent symbolism of the fig is even exalted; in fact trees usually energize men through the emission of electromagnetic waves, the Fig instead seems that steals energy from man, but it is still a theory to demonstrate.

However, the fig plant also has connotations positive; in fact, the she-wolf suckled Romulus and Remus right below to a Fico, while it was a Caprifico that prevented the two children drowned in the basket; in fact, this ran aground right below a male Fig.

The Buddha also had the lighting right under a Fig, the Ficus medica, tall about thirty meters, from whose branches hang the aerial roots that touching the ground, they give life to new trees, so the tree forms alone a grove, appearing as a kind of temple vegetable.

Ficus is part of the genus of Moraceae; the most common is the Ficus Carica or also called Female fig used in herbal medicine practice for gastritis and stomach pains, which fruits to ripen need to be fertilized by Ficus carica capricious known as Caprifico or Male an insect, the Blastophaga ensure fertilization psenes, which carries the pollen inside the inflorescences.

This is why in the past, the practice was widespread from "caprification," which consists of hanging on to the plants of Ficus carica, of the branches of Caprifico with their fruit, in period of May-June, so that the insects coming out of these carried the pollen in the real figs of the female fig.

Fig fruits are very nutritious food, rich in proteins, lipids, phosphorus, calcium, ascorbic acid trace elements. They are recommended for fatigue due to their high content of vitamins C, A, and B.

The white latex that comes out of not yet ripe fruit they favor the disappearance of corns and warts.

Returning to the Garden, there is also a wood that as we know, it has always been associated with multiple symbols.

The forest symbolizes the feminine element and the unconscious, because few rays of sunlight can penetrate for enlighten it, just as the light of reason manages to barely making unconscious contents conscious; it is expression of the dark and uncontrollable force of the nature.

In the Middle Ages, it symbolized all sorts of dangers, of threatens, being the place of ambushes, brigands, animals fierce.

And not only in a material sense but also in a sense spiritual: the forest was the negation of light, sun, and of grace; it was, in summary, the *"wild and rugged forest "*by Dante. Man is comparable to a labyrinth he risked losing his bearings and wandering indefinitely in it, prey to the dangers of him.

As if it were an initiation rite, the medieval man's life in the forest was a testing ground for forging spirit and will. The hermitage identified with the forest itself for the Western ascetic, and the hermit mimed the same fight. In ancient Rome, the Lucus was a sacred wood, distinguished by naturalness and healthiness, happy position, and climatic mildness. St. Bernard, even before that of San Francesco, had one very spiritual conception of the forest: in a letter, yes he put it this way: "In the woods, you will find something bigger than in books, trees and stones will teach you what not You will never learn from the masters. You don't think it can be sucked honey from the rocks and soil from the hardest stone?

Do not the mountains ooze sweetness and the hills of milk and honey?

Aren't the valleys covered with wheat? "And he added:" Each

I learned my knowledge of Scripture in the fields and the fields woods; beeches and oaks have always been my best masters of

God's Word. "Trees have often overgrown the role of intermediaries with the divine and occult forces.

History, tradition, classical culture often have used metaphorical concepts borrowed from the world vegetable and animal to make certain concepts clearer theorists, the story of Erisittone is an example: -Erysittone, inveterate contempt for the Gods, while he was doing cut down a forest sacred to Demeter, the Great mother of nature, it revealed itself, and since the felled trees had to serve to furnish a banquet hall; she condemned him to to be hungry forever, but a hunger so insatiable that first, he sold himself everything he owned to try to satiated, until eventually, he got to devour himself.

The moral of the story is that man destroying his mother, the Nature destroys itself.

He had many representations of the so-called Tree of Jesse, one species of the family tree built based on the Isaiah's prophecy: "A sprout will sprout from the trunk of Jesse and a branch will sprout from his roots: it will rest on him the spirit of the Lord "(Isaiah, 11,2-3). It was, therefore a allegorical tree, in which Jesse, father of the king David represented sleeping, is the root, Mary the flower and Jesus the fruit.

The passage from the Garden of Eden to the wood represents a "fall." However, the passage is deliberately represented continuously to represent the passage from a state of absolute perfection to the earthly condition.

So the arrangement of the trees within the forest is not random, in fact at the beginning you meet the trees they have preserved the memory of paradise bliss, as the Tree of Perfection and the Immortal Tree of Life, then those related to biblical or evangelical events, for example the Tree of the Cross and the Lord of the Trees, then gradually all others; however no less important in the mythological legacy a documentary of the history of humanity. A short ramp in descent out of the Garden of Eden symbolizes the fall.

At the beginning of the wood, you meet a small group of palm trees, La Palma. It has been taken as a symbol of Beauty, Perfection mathematics for the symmetry of its radius leaves, and its straight and slender stem, without branches, upwards, towards the sun. It is also a symbol of victory, rebirth, and resurrection.

In ancient Rome and Greece, it was customary to donate to the winner a palm branch, from which the expression derives

"get the palm of victory." In Greek, it was called Phoenix, as the legendary bird who lived 1461 years and it died by burning itself in its nest and then reborn from its own Ashes. Plinius reported that one existed at Cora, in lower Egypt Palma dying and spontaneously reborn; in fact, the name of this bird, phoenix, derives from the behavior of this Palma.

In Africa and the Middle East, La Palma is considered a symbol of fertility, thanks to the countless foods and drinks which offer its various species: dates, coconuts, oil, and butter obtained from the seeds of Elaeis Sinensis.

Furthermore, from the cut inflorescences of the Cocos nucifera, yes, it extracts a juice from which palm wine is obtained.

The role of Immortal Tree of Life belongs to the Cypress, which I already talked about at the beginning.

Leccio instead symbolizes the cross's Tree since it was with its wood that it was built.

A medieval legend tells that all trees do they refused to be shot down to provide wood for the cross, while il Leccio lent itself to this task, therefore apparently, Leccio takes on a connotation negative. However, if he hadn't let himself be beaten down, he wouldn't it would have been the cross and, therefore, the Redemption.

In ancient Greece, the fatal image of Leccio, in fact, was consecrated to Hecate, goddess of the underworld, while the three Fates crowned themselves with her leaves.

The Lord of the Trees instead is the Cedar, a symbol of eternity for the incorruptibility of its wood.

Of all the other trees, the Strawberry tree, characteristic of the Mediterranean scrub.

In fact, it seems that the name Conero, which gives its name to the characteristic park located in the Marche, derives from

"Komarov" strawberry tree in ancient Greek. Both the coloring and the conformation of the fruits led Pliny to consider them one species of strawberries. With the fruits of Corbezzolo, we prepare the characteristic honey indicated to combat asthma and promote diuresis. However, the Corbezzolo is to eat in moderation as it can cause serious problems intestinal. The infusion of dried leaves is antiseptic for the streets urinary tract is inflammatory for the intestine. Among the Romans, the Corbezzolo was dedicated to the goddess Carda, sister of Apollo, who with a whip of the plant she chased away witches and healed sick children, that custom was confirmed by Ovid, specifying that the children they had to be touched three times.

In the woods, there are also Acanthus trees the symbol of the resurrection is linked to the Acanthus; in fact the Acanthus leaves were adopted by Christian architecture, in Gallo-Roman capitals and in the sepulchral monuments for symbolize the Resurrection. The doctors of antiquity ne advised the infusion of leaves to calm the irritations visceral and as a preventive remedy for tuberculosis Renaissance the roots and leaves were used to obtain them emollients, poultices, and ointments.

There is also the Mistletoe that traditionally comes hung on the front door early in the year as good wish.

Mistletoe is also called St. Vitus grass, protector of people with epilepsy. In fact, both epilepsy and muscle contractions, which go by the name of San Vito dance, in tradition popular were treated with Mistletoe.

This is because, according to the theory of signature, the way of grow of the Mistletoe that never touches the ground, reports for the analogy to the fact that is treating epilepsy with Mistletoe the affected person does not fall to the ground. It is well known that the Celtic Druids collected the Mistletoe being careful not to drop it on the ground; also it they harvested with a golden sickle instead of iron.

In fact, in Bellini's "Norma" during the aria "Casta Diva," the priestess of the Druids addresses the Moon (the Casta Diva, in fact) that silver the sacred ancient plants of Mistletoe, collected by her with the golden sickle.

In the traditional pharmacopeia, the Mistletoe enjoyed great consideration as a medicinal plant: it must still be used today as a hypotensive, but should only be used on medical advice because it contains toxic substances.

In the woods, we also meet the Hawthorn, which, among other things like Mistletoe is used for high blood pressure as well for cardiac arrhythmias, as much as in traditional medicine it has earned the nickname "plant of the heart." It's great adaptability allows it to take on different shapes: round, a fan, arrow ... Make contact with a plant of Biancospino allows you to find your center and feel more serene and balanced.

Holly is a dioecious species, that is, it has both plants male and female, only the latter produce in winter red fruits, poisonous to humans but sought after by birds as winter food.

Mattioli (Sienese physician and naturalist of 1500) wrote that with its thorny fronds, it protected the salted meat from mice and other rodents: for this reason, the plant was also called Pungitopo.

At the exit of the wood is the Hortus, the cultivated countryside, the which represents the opposite of the forest; if the latter is shady and fraught with dangers, the countryside is instead sunny and reassuring, it represents tamed nature and service of man, where the forest represents nature wild and threatening.

In addition to the acquisition of the cyclical concepts of biological rhythms of plants, a medieval man related the cycles natural with the cosmic influence, and sensed a relationship with the movement of the stars, as well as hypothesizing the intervention of entities supernatural on the progress of crops.

If the Garden of Eden possessed many interpretations allegorical, in the Hortus, there are main elements of application interest.

Care for the sick was one of the main activities to which the monks dedicated themselves.

The sick were treated with medicinal plants, both with those that arose spontaneously than with those cultivated, however in the common mentality of man medieval therapeutic dynamics had to be reconciled with religious ideas of him. So Nature was seen as the source of therapeutic remedies as divine creation and proof of the Creator's goodness. The art of medicine and therapy they continued to be carried on by the monks at least until the advent of secular universities.

In 1200 the papal court aggregated to itself many scholars, including even doctors. Roger Bacon was also part of the papal circle on which posed the problem of prolonging life.

natural therefore that considered the cultural context of the court papal, even in the monasteries, the sciences were studied, if not other to the glorification of the Creator. The church was not against it to the collection and use of medicinal plants provided that remained only inside the monastery, even if in fact were also provided to external people the mastery that the monks acquired in the preparation of drugs and other natural products gave birth to a technical language appropriate to the sector.

Often it was the very appearance of the monks that inspired the name of some plants.

Medieval medical treatises were not written.

In fact, even the women had their say on the pitch doctor, in fact in the XII century, the nun Hildegard of Bingen with an intense work of correspondence, she posed at the forefront of a large group of women of the School Salernitan, some aphorisms like this have remained famous:

"If you lack doctors, let these three things be doctors:

a happy soul, rest and a moderate diet ".

The technical details for the cultivation and harvesting of herbs were also the competence of the Monacus infirmaries the need to create botanical gardens was dictated both from the need to prove from alive of the identity of medicinal plants, which for improve the safety margin in the use of herbs.

Starting from 1400, the first Herbari appeared, one a very effective tool that made the knowledge in this area. In the Middle Ages, it had great authority the encyclopedia in five volumes written by the doctor Greek Dioscorides, who also described the numerous plants exotic that he got to know through his

Chapter 8

Do you travel?

In the Middle Ages, there was also the custom of collecting plants only at certain times of the day, perhaps earlier of dawn reciting prayers, or in the period marked by a particular zodiac sign.

Pseudo-Apuleius recommended collecting the Mentastro after purifying, could you keep it in a cloth?

Clean, "and when in the baked bread, you will find a grain of whole grain, you will put it together with the Mentastro.

You will put everything under the pillow and pray to the seven planets, that is the Sun, the moon, Jupiter, Saturn, Mars, Venus, and Mercury so that in sleep, they manifest you under the protection of which one the star you are ".

Also, for the Mint, the advice was to collect it in August, before the rise of Sun.

The Betonica much praised by Augusto's doctor, yes had to collect the same in August, also there Chamomile was harvested before sunrise and after reciting the sentence: "I take you to heal the a white cloud of the pupil and for pain in the eyes, so that you can help me ".

Then it was worn around the neck closed in a bag.

For the treatment of fistulas, Agrimonia was used, of which three roots had to be collected, reciting three Paternoster e three Hail Marys After writing the patient's name on the three roots hung over a chimney and ... dried them roots, dry the fistula!

Although not all writers followed the custom of superimpose and mix pagan beliefs and myths with Christian symbolism, the phenomenon was pervasive.

As for the magical plants, it was believed that were able to operate beyond reality, whatever they were even capable of rendering invisible, immune, lucky, rich, and powerful.

The fact of aspiring to possess power prompted a fables about hypothetical plants with details powers, such as the herb Aethiopis, considered capable of drying lakes and rivers, Onothuris grass was believed to be able to open any door, while the power of driving out the enemy was the prerogative of the grass Achaemenids. It was often difficult to distinguish between the role therapeutic and magical.

Magical were those plants that had power supernatural, out of any logical explanation, to the point that Erasmus of Rotterdam defined madness as the mistress of magical herbs, in the kingdom of the Lucky Isles, where everything it was born without plowing, and the grasses flourished they stimulated the imagination: the Egyptian Lotus, the mythical Ambrosia of the Olympians, the vaunted Panacea, as well as Homeric Moly weed that I already mentioned. Some plants were surrounded from superstitions such as Lunaria, Sferracavallo. And Boris, of which it was said that the simple gesture of picking them up it would cause the storm, worship, and fear together of magical plants lasted long into the Christian era, well beyond the Middle Ages, at the end of which it seemed to explode more alive that never.

Many characters scrambled to seek power occult of plants (the elixir of life, elixir of love, the elixir of eternal youth) ...

In addition to the medicinal herb garden in the Garden, there is also the vegetable garden.

The discovery of the possibility of domestication of wild species for nutritional purposes was the point of departure for the development of agriculture and represented at the same time, a cultural turning point.

From the food point of view, the Middle Ages did not always offer food pleasant to the palate and not even of great value nutritional, which in critical periods such as during famines, it could also consist of acorns and fodder.

The importance of wheat is already attested in Roman times wheat represented and still represents the main one source of carbohydrates for many populations of the earth. La Mola the sauce was a trendy sacrificial ingredient ancient Romans, the term molar then derived from it (literally, sprinkle with mola) in the meaning of the grindstone was packed with the ears of wheat in that stage of the first formation of the embryo, stage also called latex for the tender texture of the ovary in this phase of development. The product was therefore obtained from roasting and grinding of the immature ears, just fertilized, to which salt was added collected every other day on set dates corresponding to May 8, 10, 12, 14 each year. It was not a flour of wheat but ears the specificity of the product and its use were closely connected. Indeed they identified with the cult of Ceres!

The gestural act was intended to capture the life of the grain in the its embryonic moment symbolizing the beginning creative, not so much in material as in a spiritual sense, because marked by the creative immanence of Ceres. The goddess in fact, she was the divinity of growth; she was growth itself, she was the beginning and the generation of life; hence the importance of seizing the moment of still symbolic, the Mola salsa seems who wanted to reap the fruit of the concomitant action of the primordial elements: the earth (the plant anchors its roots there and absorbs nutrients), the air (the ear is suspended there and from it absorbs light and carbon dioxide), water (plants and embryos cannot make a less, indeed they are largely constituted like all beings living) fire (understood as heat, as energy, without the which the generative act would not occur).

In many areas with a cold climate, farro was also grown and rye. But eating rye was a serious the inconvenience of Ergotism, a calamity plaguing the European populations for centuries.

In fact, in the rye, there are a parasite whose toxins released produce neurological disorders characterized by contractions and spasms of smooth muscles, which, in more cases severe leads to occlusion of the vessels in the most distal parts of the body, resulting in the stasis of circulation and necrosis of the toes and hands, if not limbs.

Only recently was the link between these bodies discovered disturbances and the intake of rye as food. Rice instead arrived in Spain with the Arabs and spread to the plains, and where there was a lot of water available. Barley so much in vogue in ancient Greece, in the Middle Ages, it lost importance and again today it is almost always used as a food As regards legumes, they were used especially lentils, peas, chickpeas, and broad beans assumed funeral connotations, connected to the Roman feast of the Lemuria: Lemurs were the wandering souls of dead people very young, who was returned to the afterlife throwing beans behind his back.

Herbs also mattered aromatic, used to make food more digestible an exploit the therapeutic properties of plants, among the species.

The most used aromatic herbs in the Middle Ages are sage, chives, horseradish, earth cress, chives, the mustard, thyme, savory, bay leaf, dill, coriander. The farmers believed that all related transactions to agriculture were mediated by influences planetary, especially from the moon, which exerts an influence magnetic, especially on plants and tides.

According to the phase the moon was in (first quarter, moon full, last quarter, new moon) were settled month by month operations such as sowing, transplanting, the fertilizing, pruning, harvesting.

Plants sown with the growing moon grow more in hurry but remain more slender, the descending moon instead favors the development of the plant in-depth, that is, the development of roots.

The therapeutic efficacy of medical herbs also changes to depending on the phase of the moon, in effect to derive the maximum therapeutic efficacy from a medicinal plant would be needed collect it at the right time that is, in the moon phase appropriate to the use you want to make of it. Many plants also open or close in operation.

The Poppy, for example, opens the flowers at six o'clock Ninfea at seven and closes them at seventeen, the Passiflora is less early in the morning; in fact, it opens daily only at noon, Calendula at nine, evening primrose at six, some Cacti a midnight.

In the medieval gardens, next to the vegetable garden, there was always the pomerium, or the orchard.

The fruit was associated with the symbol of the Cornucopia, that is the horn full of fruit and all the good things of God,

symbol of prosperity and abundance, resulting from the myth of Baby Zeus.

A fruit widely used in the Middle Ages, although it is not a real fruit is the Chestnut. The chestnut has played a fundamental role in the nutrition of the Mediterranean rural populations that it they used mainly in the form of flour proteins, lipids, iron, calcium, phosphorus, vitamin B2, and vitamin C, (however it is destroyed during cooking), so it is a nutritious and caloric fruit.

Chestnuts can have a moderate action tonic, so it can be used in decay organic, in times of stress and anemia. The real drug of the plant is contained in the leaves, which, according to the folk tradition can be used in case of whooping cough, asthmatic cough, and bronchial irritation.

The glycerine macerate of the buds instead comes used in case of varicose veins, hemorrhoids, and edema of venous origin and lymphatics of the lower limbs.

CPSIA information can be obtained
at www.ICGtesting.com
Printed in the USA
BVHW040929300421
605946BV00016B/60

9 781802 165562